Contemporary Diagnosis and Management of the Patient With Epilepsy®

Fifth Edition 2000

By

Ilo E. Leppik, MD

Director of Research, MINCEP Epilepsy Care,
Minneapolis, Minnesota

and

Clinical Professor of Neurology and Pharmacy,
University of Minnesota

Published by
Handbooks in Health Care, Newtown, Pennsylvania, USA

International Standard Book Number: 1-884065-66-x

Library of Congress Catalog Card Number: 00-01546

Contemporary Diagnosis and Management of the Patient With Epilepsy.® Copyright © 2000, 1998, 1997, 1996, 1993 by Handbooks in Health Care, a Division of AMM Co., Inc. All rights reserved. Printed in the United States of America. No part of this book may be used or reproduced in any manner whatsoever without written permission, except in the case of brief quotations embodied in critical articles and reviews. For information, write Handbooks in Health Care, 3 Terry Drive, Suite 201, Newtown, Pennsylvania 18940, 215-860-9600.
Web site: www.HHCbooks.com

Table of Contents

This book has been prepared and is presented as a service to the medical community. The information provided reflects the knowledge, experience, and personal opinions of Ilo E. Leppik, MD, Director of Research, MINCEP Epilepsy Care, and Clinical Professor of Neurology and Pharmacy, University of Minnesota, Minneapolis, Minnesota.

This book is not intended to replace or to be used as a substitute for the complete prescribing information prepared by each manufacturer for each drug. Because of possible variations in drug indications, in dosage information, in newly described toxicities, and in other items of importance, reference to such complete prescribing information is definitely recommended before any of the drugs discussed are used or prescribed.

This Fifth Edition has been extensively revised, reflecting the most current clinical developments in seizures and epilepsy.

Acknowledgments

    I would like to extend my thanks in preparing this book to Matthew T. Corso of Handbooks in Health Care Co., for his editing of the copy, and to my wife, Peggy, and our children, Peter, David, and Karina, for their patience and support.

Chapter 1

Introduction

"Epilepsy is an illness of various shapes and horrible."—Aretaeus[1]

Epilepsy and seizures are the most common serious neurologic symptoms, affecting all ages. A person experiencing a seizure and his or her family are often very frightened by seizures. Moreover, epilepsy has many socioeconomic consequences (loss of driving, social embarrassment, changes in employment). Thus, appropriate treatment must include educating the patient, counseling about emotional impact, and providing appropriate information to employers and regulatory agencies.

A critical concern to patients with epilepsy is the unpredictability of seizures; they may occur at work, while driving, or in social settings. This makes it difficult for even a person who has had only a few seizures to lead a life free of constant fear. Also, many persons are afraid of sustaining serious injury or dying during seizures, adding to their anxiety. A physician must not only prescribe medications, but must be aware of the total impact of this disorder on a person's life,

Table 1: Active Cases of Epilepsy (prevalence) per 1,000[2]	
Country	**Age-Adjusted Prevalence**
USA	
• Rochester, Minnesota	6.0
• Copiah County, Mississippi	7.0
Iceland	3.7
England	4.4
Nigeria	5.0
India (Bombay)	3.6
Guam	6.1
Poland	8.1

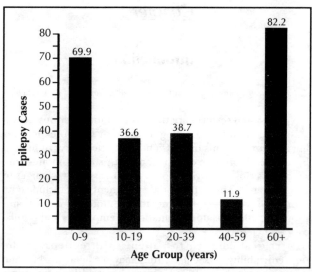

Figure 1—Histogram of average annual incidence of epilepsy by age; new cases per year per 100,000. Data from Rochester, Minnesota. Adapted from Hauser.[2]

and facilitate use of appropriate community resources to help the person with epilepsy deal effectively with this condition. Epidemiologic studies have shown that the cumulative adjusted lifetime incidence of epilepsy in Rochester, Minnesota, is 3.1% by age 80.[2] In other words, if all persons lived to age 80 in that community, 31 in 1,000 will have or have had a diagnosis of epilepsy sometime in their lives. Seizures are even more common. The lifetime cumulative incidence of seizures approaches 11%, or 110 in 1,000.[2]

Thus, most persons who experience seizures do not have epilepsy. Epilepsy is a disorder of the central nervous system (CNS) whose symptoms are seizures, but many persons will have provoked seizures (febrile convulsions, alcohol withdrawal seizures, etc) without primary CNS pathology. The clinical manifestations of a seizure, whether in a person with epilepsy or provoked, are similar, making the evaluation and treatment of a person with a single seizure particularly challenging.

The number of *active cases* (prevalence) in any given year in most countries where valid prevalence statistics are available is 5 to 8 per 1,000 (or 0.5% to 0.8%). Preliminary statistics also show that epilepsy may be more common in some underdeveloped countries (Table 1).[2] The difference between the 3.1% by age 80 incidence and the 0.5%-to-0.8% range in any given year is explained by the fact that many patients outgrow their epilepsy. The 3.1% lifetime figure includes all persons who continue to experience epileptic seizures as well as those who experienced such seizures at some time in their lives but no longer do so.

Epilepsy, by definition, is a condition in which an individual is predisposed to recurrent seizures because of a central nervous system (CNS) disorder. A seizure is a sudden, involuntary, time-limited alteration in behavior, including a change in motor activity, in autonomic function, in consciousness, or in sensation, accompanied by an abnormal electrical discharge in the brain.[3]

Many clinicians had believed that the onset of epilepsy is most common in children. But recent studies have shown that epilepsy's incidence is highest among the elderly (Figure 1).[2] One survey of nursing home residents revealed that 10.1% (4,573 of 45,405) were receiving at least one antiepileptic drug.[4]

The causes of epilepsy are many; any disease that affects the central nervous system is capable of producing epilepsy. Yet, the most common cause remains that nettlesome category, "unknown" or cryptogenic. Thus, epilepsy is not a single disease, but rather a disorder with many causes. In the young, genetic syndromes and birth trauma are the most common causes. Cerebrovascular diseases are the most common causes of epilepsy in the elderly.

Epilepsy is also variable in its degree of severity. Some persons have mild epilepsy with seizures that are completely controlled with medicine. Others continue to have a few seizures, and some patients have intractable epilepsy with multiple seizures despite appropriate treatment.

In addition, epilepsy is an episodic and paroxysmal condition. Most persons with epilepsy are completely normal between seizures, but are subject to unpredictable episodes of loss of consciousness and motor control. Thus, epilepsy is a frightening condition, misunderstood by many, including health-care professionals. This has placed an extra burden on the patient with epilepsy, who often faces discrimination in the workplace and in society.

Physicians caring for patients with epilepsy must not only have the medical knowledge to properly control seizures, but must also be sensitive to the impact this disorder has on the person as a whole. Simply controlling seizures without attending to the social and emotional issues will often lead to a less than ideal outcome.[3]

This handbook is intended to serve as an introduction to this relatively common and fascinating disorder, which can so profoundly affect the mind and consciousness.

References

1. Temkin O: *The Falling Sickness: A History of Epilepsy from the Greeks to the Beginnings of Modern Neurology.* 2nd ed, revised. Baltimore and London, Johns Hopkins Press, 1971, pp 7-9.

2. Hauser WA, Hesdorffer DC: *Epilepsy: Frequency, Causes, and Consequences.* New York, Demos Publications, 1990, pp 1-51.

3. Gumnit RJ, Leppik IE: The epilepsies. In: Rosenberg R, ed. *Comprehensive Neurology.* New York, Raven Press, 1991, pp 311-336.

4. Cloyd JC, Lackner TE, Leppik IE: Drugs in the elderly: pharmacoepidemiology and pharmacokinetics. *Arch Fam Med* 1994;3:589-598.

Chapter 2

Seizures

Over the ages, many different terms have been used to describe epilepsy and seizures. This proliferation of descriptive words has led to unnecessary confusion among patients and health-care providers. This chapter will review the terminology and classification of seizures; in Chapter 3 we will examine the classification of the epileptic syndromes.

The word *seizure* is sometimes used vaguely to refer to a sudden, catastrophic event, especially if the precise nature of the event is unknown. Many other words have been used in this context, including *fit*, *spell*, and *attack*. In this handbook, a seizure is defined as a paroxysmal, time-limited event that results from abnormal neuronal activity in the brain. However, physicians may face a situation in which the precise nature of the event being evaluated has not been determined. In this circumstance, 'possible seizure' would be a better description to avoid labeling someone before a definitive diagnosis is made.

Most seizures are not epileptic (nonepileptic), that is, not generated primarily by the brain. Nonepileptic seizures may be either physiologic or psychogenic. Nonepileptic physiologic seizures are a response to some disturbance external to the central nervous system, such as hypoxia, toxins, or fever (Figure 1). Nonepileptic psychogenic seizures are often a reaction to psychic stress. Epileptic seizures can arise from distinct regions of the brain (localization-related), or be caused by a general dysfunction of the biochemical mechanisms (generalized).

Behavioral Features

The major behavioral features of seizures that distinguish them from usual activity are that they are stereotypical and repetitive. They lack the typical modulation seen with volitional behavior. For example, a clonic seizure involves maximal contraction of skeletal muscles, followed by relaxation, with the cycle usually repeated a few times per second. This very primitive movement pattern accomplishes no useful func-

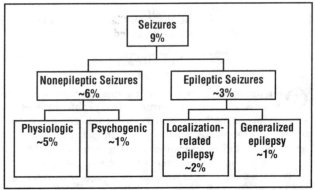

Figure 1—Subdivision of seizures into etiologic categories and their appropriate lifetime incidences.

tion and is in marked contrast to the usual complex, modulated activity that our muscle groups are capable of performing.

Generalized tonic-clonic seizures can evolve from partial seizures (**I** C in Table 1) or can be generalized from the onset (**II** E in Table 1). Although generalized tonic-clonic seizures of either type are indistinguishable in the clinical setting, it is critical for appropriate treatment that the correct classification be made.

More common than the dramatic generalized tonic-clonic seizures (GTS) are the partial seizures. These may be simple or complex and may evolve into secondarily generalized tonic-clonic seizures (Table 1). In 1954, Penfield used the term *automatism* to describe the unconscious, meaningless behavior exhibited by persons having a complex partial seizure.[1] A patient with complex partial seizures may perform activities that superficially appear normal, but that are done without seeming comprehension of the social setting. For example, one of my patients was described by his friends as experiencing the following: while playing cards, he developed a blank look on his face, put down his cards, walked slowly to the refrigerator, opened its door, urinated, and then appeared confused. Upon recovering awareness, he had no recollection of this event. Fortunately, his friends were aware of his epilepsy, and had seen other episodes of his unusual behavior. Imagine the re-

Table 1: Epileptic Seizures: Classification and Characteristics, as Proposed by the ILAE[2]

I. Partial Seizures (Focal Seizures)

A. Simple partial seizures
   1. with motor signs
   2. with somatosensory or special sensory symptoms
   3. with autonomic symptoms
   4. with psychic symptoms

B. Complex partial seizures
   1. simple partial onset followed by impairment of consciousness
   2. with impairment of consciousness at the onset

C. Partial seizures evolving to secondarily generalized seizures
   1. simple partial seizures
      (a) evolving to generalized seizures
   2. complex partial seizures
      (b) evolving to generalized seizures
   3. simple partial seizures evolving to complex partial seizures evolving to generalized seizures

II. Generalized Seizures (Convulsive or Nonconvulsive)

A. 1. typical absence seizures (*petit mal*)
   2. atypical
B. Myoclonic seizures
C. Clonic seizures
D. Tonic seizures
E. Tonic-clonic seizures (*grand mal*)
F. Atonic seizures

III. Unclassified Epileptic Seizures

• Includes all those seizures that cannot be classified because of incomplete data or because they defy classification into the above catagories; for example, neonatal seizures with swimming movements.

IV. Status Epilepticus

Used with permission, *Epilepsia 1981;22:489-501.*

action to this behavior from persons not familiar with the manifestations of complex partial seizures.

One of the major developments in epileptology has been the adoption of the International Classification of Epileptic

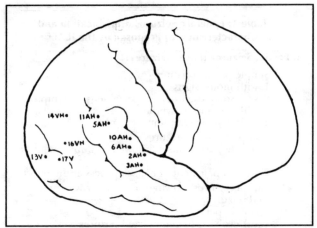

Figure 2—*Classic depiction of partial stimulation record. V=visual response; VH=visual hallucinatory seizure; AH=auditory hallucinatory seizure. Reprinted with permission from* Epilepsy and the Functional Anatomy of the Human Brain. *1st ed. Boston, Little, Brown and Co, 1954, p 464.*

Seizures (ICES).[2] At the core of this scheme, illustrated in Table 1, is the recognition of two major categories of seizures: those that begin locally in a specific region of the brain and then spread (partial seizures), and those that are generalized at onset (generalized seizures). Much of the basis for this classification is the recognition that the brain is highly organized, with specific functions represented in discrete anatomical regions. Thus, epileptic seizures that have their genesis in a discrete region of the brain (focus) are classified as partial seizures (Table 1). Conversely, those seizures for which there is no identifiable focal origin are classified as generalized. This division by physiologic criteria has proven useful in understanding epilepsy and in determining therapeutic strategies. This concept was elegantly discussed in a seminal book, *Epilepsy and the Functional Anatomy of the Human Brain*, by Penfield and Jasper.[1] This work was important in our understanding of the brain's organization (Figure 2). Their book provides numerous case reports of patients who had epilepsy surgery under local anesthesia, and those patients' responses to direct

Table 2: Summary of Clinical and EEG Features of Epileptic Seizures

Seizure	Usual Duration	Loss of Consciousness	Postseizure Confusion	EEG During Seizure
Simple partial	5-10 sec	no	no	normal or focal spikes
Complex partial	variable; 5-10 sec, 1-2 min, 5+ min rarely	yes	yes	focal activity spreading to involve one or both hemispheres
Absence	5-10 sec, may cluster	yes	no	generalized, 3 per second, spike and wave
Generalized tonic clonic-	1-2 min	yes	yes	series of generalized, high-amplitude spikes

cortical stimulation. This stimulation was done both to identify the function of the cortex, which might need to be surgically removed, and relate it to the focus or site of onset of a patient's seizure.

In addition to clinical features, the electroencephalograph (EEG) is essential in classifying seizures: partial seizures have focal discharges, while generalized seizures have abnormalities over all head regions at onset (Table 2).

Simple Partial Seizures

The partial seizures are further subdivided by their effect on consciousness. Seizures in which consciousness is not altered are termed simple. An example of a simple partial seizure is a feeling such as that of a breeze over an extremity. "Aura" is the original Greek word for breeze, and was described in the medical writings of Hippocrates as the first sensation felt by a young man just before he was stricken with a generalized tonic-clonic seizure.[3] We now know that the origin of this kind of seizure is in the somatosensory area of the brain, contralateral to the limb experiencing the feeling. This simple partial seizure may progress into a secondarily generalized tonic-clonic seizure. Using the old terminology, this patient would be described as having an *aura*, followed by a *grand mal* seizure. The Jacksonian seizure is one in which a patient has clonic activity, usually involving the hand, contralateral to a lesion in the motor cortex, which progresses to a generalized tonic-clonic seizure.

The only difference between a Jacksonian seizure and a grand mal seizure preceded by a sensory aura is the location of the focus, but this similarity is not easily deduced from the old terminology. Furthermore, seizure manifestations change with medical treatment, so that often a person with Jacksonian seizures may no longer experience generalized tonic-clonic seizures with treatment, but still have brief motor seizures or "minor motor" seizures by the old classification system.

Simple motor seizures (**I.** A.1. in Table 1) arise from the motor cortex (frontal lobe). Usually, they consist of rapid clonic activity. Sometimes they may be rapid jerks, and the EEG spikes are time-locked to EMG silence.[4] Other simple motor seizures are those with versive or postural movements. Simple partial seizures may have somatosensory phenomena (feeling of a breeze), visual (light flashes, formed visual hallucinations), visual distortions such as macropsia (things appear large), auditory (buzzing), olfactory, gustatory, and vertiginous symptoms. Autonomic symptoms include epigastric rising sensation (described by some as the feeling one gets going down a roller coaster), sweating, flushing, piloerection, and pupillary dilatation. Psychic symptoms include fear, anger, dreamy states, and the classic déjà vu ("I've seen this before") sensation.

These events are sometimes difficult to separate from psychological phenomena. The two key features of epileptic seizures that distinguish them from the manifestations of psychiatric disorders are that seizures occur paroxysmally, that is, without warning and without preceding provocative events, and that they occur in patients who are relatively free of significant psychiatric disorders. Also of help is the fact that most simple partial seizures last less than a minute (Table 2). Sometimes, however, it can be difficult to determine whether a patient has had a panic attack or a simple partial psychic seizure, and the treatments are quite different.

Complex Partial Seizures

Complex partial seizures involve impairment or loss of consciousness. Loss or alteration of consciousness in epilepsy does not refer to coma; rather, a lack of understanding and memory of the event is implied. As Penfield[1] explained: "The state in which an individual is able to move about in a relatively normal manner but is, at the same time, suddenly lacking in understanding is called automatism. Subsequently, he will have amnesia for the period. He may seem to be an automaton and yet is sometimes partially receptive of direction from others." This implies alteration of functioning in the mesial temporal lobes, in the orbitofrontal lobes, or in more widespread areas of the brain. Complex partial seizures in the past have been referred to as *psychomotor seizures*, but this term is vague and ill-defined. They have been called temporal lobe seizures and they can originate from extratemporal structures.

Complex partial seizures may last a few seconds. These brief episodes may be confused with absence seizures, and not infrequently may be called "petit mal." In the past, some referred to these as temporal lobe absence seizures. However, a clear distinction must be made because medications used for absence seizures are not effective for complex partial seizures. Most complex partial seizures last for 1 to 3 minutes, sometimes longer. Patients usually experience a period of confusion after the seizure, lasting for a few minutes. Patients cannot recall any of the events that occurred during the seizure.

The automatism has no lateralizing value. For example, one right-handed patient snapped his fingers during an automatism, yet his focus was in the right temporal lobe. Sometimes complicated behaviors occur during a complex partial seizure. These often involve partial undressing, urination, or other socially embarrassing behavior, of which the patient with epilepsy has no recall after the seizure. "Cursive epilepsy," characterized by frantic running, and "gelastic epilepsy," characterized by uncontrollable laughing, are complex seizures and are classified under **I. B.1.** or **I. B.2.** (Table 1), depending on onset.

Secondarily Generalized Tonic-Clonic Seizures

Any partial seizure can generalize into a tonic-clonic seizure. Indeed, patients with partial seizures rarely present initially to the medical system for their partial seizures. Instead, they are often brought to the hospital emergency department after an unrecognized and untreated partial seizure generalizes and the patient experiences a generalized tonic-clonic *(grand mal)* seizure. Clinicians must be careful not to assume from the outset that a seizure was generalized. Most generalized tonic-clonic seizures in adults are secondarily generalized, or I.C., seizures.

Primary Generalized Seizures

Primary generalized seizures can be convulsive, that is, tonic-clonic *(grand mal)*, or nonconvulsive. Absence seizures are what many have called "petit mal" in the past. In medieval France, the term "grand mal," literally translated as the big sickness, was used to designate a great epileptic attack. In contrast, the term "petit mal" or little sickness was used to describe a small seizure. The terms *grand mal* and *petit mal* are no longer specific enough to be useful in contemporary usage.

Absence seizures are most common in childhood. They are manifested by impairment of consciousness, eye blinking, staring, and other minor facial movements. They last from a few seconds to a minute. However, they may occur many times a day in rapid succession. An important consequence is the time lost, with the result that many children often have poor school performance. (These are described in more detail in Chapter 3.)

Myoclonic seizures consist of quick muscle jerks. These may be bilateral or unilateral and are usually seen in specific epilepsy syndromes. Consciousness is not usually impaired. However, myoclonic activity may also be associated with other neurologic disorders (Creutzfeldt-Jakob disease, anoxia). Furthermore, it may be difficult to readily categorize myoclonus.

Tonic seizures consist of tonic spasms of truncal and facial muscles associated with flexion of upper extremities and extension of lower extremities. They are most common in childhood and may result in falls.

Clonic seizures are most common in children, and may resemble myoclonus except that there is a loss of consciousness and that the repetition rate is slower than in myoclonus.

Tonic-clonic seizures are the most dramatic of all seizure types. Generalized tonic-clonic seizures begin suddenly, without warning. (If the patient reports an "aura," the event was most likely a partial seizure with secondary generalization). Typically, the patient cries out as tonic contraction of the trunk muscles forces expiration. The generalized tonic phase then becomes interrupted by short periods of relaxation followed by tonic contractions. Then, the periods of relaxation become more frequent and the clonic phase begins. The seizure is accompanied by a marked increase in heart rate and blood pressure. The seizures last 1 to 2 minutes. Occasionally, they may occur in rapid succession and become status epilepticus. After the seizure is over, incontinence may occur as the sphincter muscles relax. Not all tonic-clonic seizures are followed by incontinence. Full consciousness might not return for 10 to 15 minutes, and confusion and fatigue may persist for hours or days.

Atonic seizures are characterized by the patient suddenly dropping to the floor from a loss of tone in postural muscles. Atonic seizures are most commonly seen in children with the Lennox-Gastaut syndrome. The attacks generally last only a few seconds and can occur without any loss of consciousness. However, these seizures are dangerous because they have a high rate of injury from falls. It is often difficult to distinguish between atonic and tonic seizures.

References

1. Penfield W, Jasper H: *Epilepsy and the Functional Anatomy of the Human Brain*. Boston, Little, Brown and Co, 1954, p 27.

2. Commission on Classification and Terminology of the International League Against Epilepsy. Proposal for revised clinical and electroencephalographic classification of epileptic seizures. *Epilepsia* 1981;22:489-501.

3. Temkin O: *The Falling Sickness: A History of Epilepsy from the Greeks to the Beginnings of Modern Neurology*. 2nd ed, revised. Baltimore and London, Johns Hopkins Press, 1971, pp 28-50.

4. Guerrini R, Dravet C, Genton P, et al: Epileptic negative myoclonus. *Neurology* 1993;43:1078-1083.

Selected Reading

Engel J Jr: *Seizures and Epilepsy*. Philadelphia, FA Davis Co, 1989.

Chapter 3

Epilepsy and the Epileptic Syndromes

Epilepsy is a disorder of the central nervous system (CNS) whose symptoms are seizures. The clinician must try to determine the underlying epileptic syndrome because this has profound implications for treatment and prognosis.[1] In other words, the seizure is a nonspecific symptom of a disorder that must be further diagnosed. This is analogous to fever being the symptom of any number of disease processes. To help organize the diagnosis of the underlying disorder, the International League Against Epilepsy (ILAE) has developed a classification of the epilepsies and epileptic syndromes (Table 1).[2] Many of these syndromes have age-specific onset and clinical characteristics that have been clearly delineated (Table 2).

The first step in identifying the epileptic syndrome is correctly identifying the type of seizure that a person has.[3] An epileptic syndrome may include more than one seizure type. For example, a patient can have both simple partial motor and secondarily generalized tonic-clonic seizures (types **I.** A.1. and **I.**C. as listed in Table 1, Chapter 2), but only one syndrome (case 1 at end of this chapter). Or, a person with the syndrome of juvenile myoclonic epilepsy has absence, myoclonic, and generalized tonic-clonic seizures (types **II.** A.1., **II.** B., and **II.** E.). Consequently, physicians must consider a number of factors when attempting to identify a patient's epileptic syndrome (Table 3).

In the ILAE's classification system of the epilepsies, the primary distinction is based on the patient's seizure type, either partial or generalized. Thus, the fundamental distinction is between the localization-related versus the generalized epilepsies. Localization-related epileptic syndromes are often caused by identifiable lesions, whereas the generalized epileptic syndromes are *idiopathic*.

Many causes of epilepsy have been identified. Epilepsies associated with CNS pathology are labeled secondary or symptomatic. If the etiology is unknown, the term *cryp-*

Table 1: International Classification of Epilepsies and Epileptic Syndromes

1. **Localization-Related (Focal, Local, Partial) Epilepsies and Syndromes**

    1.1 Idiopathic with age-related onset
    At present, two syndromes are established, but more may be identified in the future:
    - Benign childhood epilepsy with centrotemporal spikes
    - Childhood epilepsy with occipital paroxysms

    1.2 Symptomatic
    This category comprises syndromes of great individual variability, which will mainly be based on anatomical localization, clinical features, seizure types, and etiological factors. Epileptic syndromes of unknown etiology are classified as cryptogenic.

2. **Generalized Epilepsies and Syndromes**

    2.1 Idiopathic, with age-related onset, listed in order of age
    - Benign neonatal familial convulsions
    - Benign neonatal convulsions
    - Benign myoclonic epilepsy in infancy
    - Childhood absence epilepsy (pyknolepsy)
    - Juvenile absence epilepsy
    - Juvenile myoclonic epilepsy (impulsive petit mal)
    - Epilepsy with grand mal seizures on awakening

    Other generalized idiopathic epilepsies, if they do not belong to one of the above syndromes, can still be classified as generalized idiopathic epilepsies.

    2.2 Idiopathic and/or symptomatic, in order of age of appearance
    - West's syndrome (infantile spasms)
    - Lennox-Gastaut syndrome
    - Epilepsy with myoclonic-astatic seizures
    - Epilepsy with myoclonic absences

(continued on next page)

Table 1 *(continued)*

2.3 Symptomatic

    2.3.1   Nonspecific etiology
         - Early myoclonic encephalopathy

    2.3.2   Specific syndromes
         - Epileptic seizures may complicate many disease states.
         - Included under this heading are those diseases in which seizures are a presenting or predominant feature.

3. Epilepsies and Syndromes Undetermined as to Whether They Are Focal or Generalized

3.1 With both generalized and focal seizures
- Neonatal seizures
- Severe myoclonic epilepsy in infancy
- Epilepsy with continuous spike waves during slow wave sleep
- Acquired epileptic aphasia (Landau-Kleffner syndrome)

3.2 Without unequivocal generalized or focal features

This heading covers all cases where clinical and EEG findings do not permit classification as clearly generalized or localization-related, such as in many cases of sleep grand mal.

4. Special Syndromes

4.1 Situation-related seizures
- Febrile convulsions
- Seizures related to other identifiable situations such as stress, hormonal changes, drugs, alcohol, or sleep deprivation

4.2 Isolated, apparently unprovoked epileptic events

4.3 Epilepsies characterized by specific modes of seizure precipitation

4.4 Chronic progressive epilepsia partialis continua of childhood

Used with permission, *Epilepsia 1989;30:389-399.*

togenic is used; otherwise, the cause is listed, ie, symptomatic epilepsy secondary to stroke. Epilepsies occurring without CNS pathology are labeled primary or idiopathic. Inherent in the classification is the notion that the primary,

Table 2: Pediatric Epilepsy Syndromes by Age of Onset

Newborns

- Benign neonatal convulsions (fifth-day fits)
- Familial benign neonatal convulsions
- Early myoclonic encephalopathy
- Severe idiopathic status epilepticus
- Early infantile epileptic encephalopathy with suppression-burst

Infants

- Febrile convulsions
- West's syndrome: Infantile spasms
- Benign myoclonic epilepsy in infants
- Severe myoclonic epilepsy in infants
- Myoclonic epilepsy (myoclonic status) in nonprogressive encephalopathies
- Epileptic seizures caused by inborn errors of metabolism
- Myoclonic-astatic epilepsy of early childhood
- Lennox-Gastaut syndrome

Children

- Childhood absence epilepsy (pyknolepsy)
- Epilepsy with myoclonic absences
- Epilepsy with generalized convulsive seizures
- Benign partial epilepsies
- Benign epilepsy with centrotemporal (rolandic) spikes (BERS)
- Benign psychomotor epilepsy
- Benign epilepsy with occipital spike-waves (BEOSW)
- Other benign partial epilepsies
- Benign partial epilepsy with extreme somatosensory-evoked potentials
- Landau-Kleffner syndrome
- Epilepsy with continuous spikes and waves during sleep
- Epilepsy with photosensitivity
- Eyelid myoclonia absences
- Self-induced epilepsy

(continued on next page)

Table 2 *(continued)*

Older Children and Adolescents (Juveniles)

- Juvenile absence epilepsy
- Juvenile myoclonic epilepsy (JME)
- Epilepsy with grand mal on awakening (GMA)
- Benign partial seizures of adolescence
- Kojewnikoff's syndrome
- Progressive myoclonus epilepsies
  - Juvenile Gaucher's
  - Juvenile neuronal ceroid lipofuscinosis (NCL)
  - Lafora's body disease
- Unverricht-Lundborg disease (Finnish or Baltic myoclonus epilepsy)
  - Cherry-red spot myoclonus (neuraminidase deficiency)
  - Dyssynergia cerebellaris myoclonica (Ramsay Hunt syndrome)
  - Mitochondrial encephalopathy

idiopathic epilepsies have strong genetic foundations and recent discoveries have linked specific gene defects and gene products, including the human GABA BR1 receptor, with these syndromes.[2,4,5] Idiopathic or primary forms of the various epilepsies usually carry a better prognosis for response to treatment and possible remission than the secondary epilepsies.

The proper classification of seizures is of great value in helping localize the brain regions involved. But identifying the correct type of seizure is not necessarily useful in determining the underlying pathology. For example, when evaluating a patient with simple partial motor seizures involving the left hand, the clinician can deduce that there is a lesion in the right motor cortex hand area. However, one cannot determine if the lesion is a tumor, an arteriovenous malformation, cysticercosis, or a cerebral cicatrix (scar) from an old injury. Other studies are needed to determine the pathology, but knowledge of the site can help guide diagnostic studies.

Table 3: Factors to Identify the Epileptic Syndrome

- Seizure type(s)
- EEG (ictal and interictal)
- Etiology
- MRI scan
- Response to AEDs
- Inheritance
- Natural history

Localization-Related
(Focal, Local, Partial) Epilepsies (1)

Localization-related epilepsies are described as either idiopathic or symptomatic. In the idiopathic (possibly genetic) category, only a few specific syndromes have been identified, appearing in childhood and with specific clinical and EEG features. On the other hand, there are numerous symptomatic epilepsies.

Idiopathic (1.1)

Benign epilepsy of childhood with centrotemporal spikes (BECTS, Rolandic epilepsy) is a common syndrome, and may account for as many as one quarter of epilepsy cases in school-aged children.[6] It has its onset between ages 3 and 13. The seizures have a simple partial onset, usually beginning in the face and variably generalizing to tonic-clonic seizures. The seizures occur almost always at night.[7] The children have normal neurological examinations and no associated illnesses. The EEG findings are classic and consist of high-amplitude spikes and sharp waves in the central region, which are most frequent during light sleep. The EEG findings are so diagnostic that many pediatric neurologists feel that structural studies such as magnetic resonance imaging (MRI) are unnecessary. Etiology is genetic, with an autosomal dominant inheritance reported for the EEG trait, but less than 25% of patients with the EEG pattern actually develop seizures.[8] A recent study demonstrated a link between chromosome 15q14 and families with BECTS.[9] Prognosis is excellent; seizures are easily controlled with carbamazepine, phenytoin, or gabapentin and almost all children outgrow these without sequelae by age 15.[10]

**Table 4: Some Causes of Symptomatic
Localization-Related Epilepsies**

Vascular
- stroke
- infantile hemiplegia
- arteriovenous
  malformations
- Sturge-Weber syndrome
- aneurysms (subarachnoid
  hemorrhage)
- venous thrombosis
- hypertensive
  encephalopathy
- blood dyscrasias
  (sickle cell anemia)

Infectious
- abscess
- meningitis and encephalitis
- toxoplasmosis
- rubella
- Rasmussen's syndrome
  (presumed viral)
- cysticercosis

Tumors
- meningiomas
- gliomas
- hamartomas
- metastatic tumors

Degenerative
- Alzheimer's
- multiple sclerosis

Congenital
- heterotopias
- cortical dysplasias

Traumatic
- prenatal and
  perinatal injuries
- head injuries

Cryptogenic
- no cause identified

Childhood epilepsy with occipital spikes is much less common; it is characterized by daytime seizures consisting of visual experiences followed by complex partial seizures. After the seizure, patients often have a headache. The EEG shows bilateral, high-amplitude spike-and-wave discharges in the occipital region; the course is benign.

Symptomatic (1.2)

Symptomatic localization-related epilepsies are the most common syndrome in adults and have many specific identifiable causes (Table 4). Despite the large number of causes in this category, seizure types are limited to partial seizures that often, if untreated, progress to secondarily generalized tonic-clonic seizures. Thus, the phenomenology of the seizure is helpful in directing attention to the fact that identifiable and potentially treatable pathology is present, but is not helpful in identifying the etiology, which must be done by the diagnostic evaluation. The underlying pathology may be diffuse or multifocal, such as anoxia, physical trauma (head injury), or infections. Other causes are more focal, such as cerebrovascular disease (stroke, arteriovenous malformations, subarachnoid hemorrhage, venous thrombosis), brain tumors (astrocytomas, meningiomas, glioblastomas, metastatic tumors), and mesial temporal sclerosis. Mesial temporal sclerosis may be one of the most surgically treatable of the epilepsies and will be discussed more fully in Chapter 13.

However, despite careful history-taking and the use of improved diagnostic techniques, in many cases the cause of the epilepsy cannot be determined. These are classified as cryptogenic. Consequently, epilepsy of undetermined origin or *symptomatic cryptogenic* is still the most common "syndrome" in this category. However, with high-resolution MRI scans, cortical heterotopias (migrational defects) are now being recognized in many patients with intractable *cryptogenic* epilepsy.

Generalized Epilepsies and Syndromes (2)

The generalized epilepsies are most common in the pediatric population. Idiopathic (genetic) syndromes have been well defined in the last few years, and indeed, gene foci have been mapped for some, cementing firmly the concept of a specific identifiable syndrome.

Idiopathic with Age-Related Onset (2.1)

Benign neonatal familial convulsions is a rare syndrome characterized by generalized seizures occurring only during the first week of life. It must be differentiated from the long list of more serious symptomatic neonatal seizures. There is usually a clear family history and the seizures remit spontaneously after a few days. A deletion of chromosome 20q13.3 has been identified, and DNA of this region encodes a potassium channel, thus providing a clear relationship between a gene product and clinical syndrome.[11] Another infrequent disorder, benign myoclonic epilepsy in infancy, is differentiated in this age group by an EEG with bursts of spike-and-wave discharges superimposed on an otherwise normal background.

Childhood Absence (Pyknolepsy) was referred to as "petit mal epilepsy" in the past. However, because of the wide misuse of the term petit mal, the more accurate term of childhood absence has been applied to this condition. The term pyknolepsy (pyknos refers to crowding) is also used to describe this condition[12] because seizures have a tendency to occur many times an hour. They consist of the typical absence seizures described in Chapter 2. Although each seizure may be short, the fact that these seizures occur in rapid succession often leads to considerable dysfunction because of the time the child loses from school and other learning activities. The EEG is characterized by the classical 3-per-second spike-and-wave discharge occurring on an otherwise normal background.[13] Structural studies are usually not indicated. Childhood absence epilepsy occurs in 2% to 4% of children with epilepsy. The major differential diagnosis of this staring behavior is brief partial complex seizures.

Childhood absence epilepsy remits in 40% of patients, so lifelong therapy may not be needed.[3] The two drugs that are most effective in absence epilepsy are ethosuximide and valproate. Because childhood absence epilepsy is benign, ethosuximide is recommended first; valproate is recommended when ethosuximide is insufficient or when the patient also has generalized tonic-clonic seizures. However, some may have generalized tonic-clonic seizures that persist into later life. There is a strong genetic predisposition, and a specific gene locus is suspected.

Juvenile myoclonic epilepsy (JME) has its onset during the teenage years and is a characteristic syndrome consisting of a triad of seizures (myoclonic, absence, and generalized tonic-clonic). Myoclonic seizures usually occur in the morning and involve primarily the upper extremities. The most common complaint is clumsiness or jitters, which is exacerbated by stress and is often initially mistaken for adolescent behavior. Generalized tonic-clonic seizures develop, usually in the morning. Absence seizures may be relatively difficult to detect. Not all persons have all three seizure types, but the EEG characteristics along with the history are usually diagnostic. It is important to differentiate this syndrome from localization-related epilepsies because treatment is highly specific; response to carbamazepine or phenytoin is usually poor, while valproate is very effective. A specific gene locus in chromosome 6p21.2-p11 has been proposed for this familial syndrome.[14]

Symptomatic and/or Idiopathic (2.2)

This group of generalized epilepsy consists of a mixed set of clinical syndromes. What unites them in the classification is that their clinical manifestations are similar. Some children in these groups have identifiable symptomatic causes, while in others the etiology is undetermined, or cryptogenic. Unlike category 2.1 (Table 1), in which seizures occur in the setting of normal intelligence as the sole manifestation of the syndrome, in this group mental retardation is common.

Infantile spasms, also known as West's syndrome or salaam seizures, begin between the ages of 4 and 12 months. It is defined by a specific seizure type, a spasm that consists of flexion at the neck, waist, arms, and legs, with either abduction or adduction of the arms. These are quick, lasting only a second, hence the name "blitzkrampf," or lightning seizure. These may occur hundreds of times a day. Infants with this syndrome usually develop normally until spasms occur, at which point there is arrest of psychomotor development. Approximately two thirds of patients have an EEG pattern described as hypsarrhythmia and one third have large definable abnormalities. The hypsarrhythmia pattern is a disorganized mixture of spikes and slow waves that are different in each hemisphere.

The prognosis in infantile spasms is related to the underlying brain disorder and to the therapy.[15] Patients with idiopathic infantile spasms who respond to optimal therapy have the best prognosis. Those with severe encephalopathic disorders have the worst. Among all patients with infantile spasms, 20% die before 5 years of age, and of the survivors between 75% and 93% are reported to be mentally retarded; up to 50% have epilepsy later in life, and half of these develop the Lennox-Gastaut syndrome.

Current therapy of infantile spasms is adrenocorticotrophic hormone (ACTH) initiated within 1 month of the onset of spasms. This is associated with 5% mortality from complications of therapy, most often overwhelming infection.[16] When ACTH and steroids are ineffective, conventional anticonvulsants are used, most often a benzodiazepine such as clonazepam. Recently, vigabatrin has been reported to be particularly effective for control of seizures if West's syndrome is caused by tuberous sclerosis.

27

Lennox-Gastaut syndrome has been designated to represent a combination of seizures—axial tonic attacks, tonic-clonic seizures, atypical absence seizures, and atonic or so-called drop attacks—with mental subnormality and an EEG pattern of slow (< 2.5 Hz) spike and wave.[17,18] Onset is between 1 to 8 years. Lennox-Gastaut syndrome is typically difficult to treat. Valproate, benzodiazepines, and felbamate are most effective,[19] but some of the other drugs sometimes actually worsen the akinetic and atypical absence seizures.

Epilepsies, Undetermined as to Focal or Generalized (3)

In this category of epilepsies are a number of pediatric syndromes (Tables 1 and 2) whose clinical natures have not yet been fully elucidated. Some patients may experience a mixture of focal and generalized EEG patterns and clinical seizures. This group includes a number of cases of myoclonic epilepsy with mental retardation.

Special Syndromes (4)

This category is designed to encompass conditions in which seizures do not occur spontaneously, but rather are related to specific stimuli. Thus, these patients probably have some predisposing CNS dysfunction. However, unlike the epileptic syndromes described above, treatment for these special conditions often consists of avoiding the specific stimuli, or treating only at the time of provocation. Also in this group are patients who have isolated seizures and may simply have a low seizure threshold.

Situation-Related Seizures

Febrile seizures (febrile convulsions) occur among children from 3 months of age to 5 years of age who have fever and no evidence of another cause. Although their reported incidence varies, in one large study these seizures occurred in 4.2% of black children and 3.5% of white children.[20] A family history of febrile seizures was present in 8% to 22% of parents and in 9% to 17% of siblings of the patient. This study found that offspring of febrile seizure patients had an 11% chance of having this kind of seizure. A specific linkage to

> ### Table 5: Factors in Febrile Seizures Associated With Increased Risk of Epilepsy at Age 7 Years[18]
>
> - Family history of later epilepsy
> - Preexisting neurologic abnormality
> - Complex febrile seizure
>   > 15 minutes duration
>   > 1 febrile seizure per 24 h
> - Focal febrile seizure
>
> Used with permission, *Pediatrics 1978;61:720-727.*

chromosome 19q13.1, which may code for a mutation in the voltage-gated sodium channel beta1 subunit, has been reported in some families with febrile seizures, but there may be other genes in other families.[21]

Prospective population-based studies indicate that febrile seizures are relatively benign.[22,23] Febrile seizures are not associated with an increased risk of mental retardation or of serious neurologic impairment. Overall, the chance of epilepsy after febrile seizures is small, with 3% developing epilepsy by 7 years of age and approximately 7% by 25 years of age.[20,23,24] Epilepsy is more likely to appear when certain risk factors are present (Table 5).

The risk of additional febrile seizures is related to the patient's age at the time of the first febrile seizure. Overall, the risk of recurrence is 34%, although it is higher in younger children. Among those patients who have their first febrile seizure before the age of 12 months, the chance of a second seizure is 50%. For this reason, some authorities recommend initiating treatment for children with febrile seizures who are less than 18 months old.[25]

Treatment is controversial; many pediatric neurologists do not recommend chronic treatment for simple febrile seizures. The side effects of phenobarbital, mainly adverse behavior, are expected in up to 40% of patients. Slight cognitive side effects of phenobarbital also offset potential benefits.[26] In Europe, diazepam per rectum is given when fever occurs to prevent febrile convulsions.[27-29] A rectal diazepam product is available in the United States (Rectal Diastat®), and is approved by the FDA for use against acute repetitive seizures but not febrile convulsions.[30]

Case Reports

When treating a patient with epilepsy, it is important to classify not only the seizure type, but also the epilepsy syndrome. As the following case histories demonstrate, doing so leads to a specific treatment plan and prognostic information.

Case 1: The parents of an 8-year-old boy were aroused one night by noise from his bedroom. When they rushed to his room they saw the bedsheets awry and their son breathing deeply. He appeared to have bitten his tongue. In the emergency department he was mildly confused, afebrile, and had a lacerated tongue. He was admitted for observation, and an EEG the next day showed centrotemporal spikes. No further tests were done and he was discharged on no medications after discussion with his parents. However, a second nocturnal seizure occurred a year later and he was given medication. He was treated until age 12, when the medication was discontinued.

Seizure type: secondarily generalized tonic-clonic (**I.C**)

Epileptic syndrome: benign childhood epilepsy with centrotemporal spikes

Etiology: idiopathic

Prognosis: spontaneous remission with maturity

Case 2: A 36-year-old, right-handed construction worker had been suffering from pounding headaches, often brought on by exertion, for about 1 year. He also noticed that he did not seem to have the strength and coordination in his left hand that he was accustomed to having. Also, he occasionally found that his left hand would "jerk" for a few seconds. This became progressively worse, but he did not seek medical attention until he had a generalized tonic-clonic seizure at home. He was admitted to St. Paul-Ramsey Medical Center in St. Paul, Minnesota, for evaluation and treatment. A CT scan showed a vascular lesion in the right frontal region extending to the motor area. A CT scan with contrast demonstrated this to be an arteriovenous malformation (AVM). He was initially treated with phenobarbital and phenytoin. Consideration was given to surgery, but it was deemed too risky because of the AVM's large size and its involvement of the motor area. He has been well controlled for the last 12 years in that he has not had any more generalized tonic-clonic seizures, but he continues to have periodic simple partial seizures. He also continues to have intermittent headaches and has had some mild decrease of function in the left hand.

Seizure types: simple partial seizures with motor symptoms (**I.** A.1) and secondarily generalized tonic-clonic seizures (**I. C**)

Epileptic syndrome: localization-related symptomatic (1.2)

Etiology: arteriovenous malformation

Prognosis: lifelong risk for seizures with possible worsening of motor dysfunction and intracerebral hemorrhage from AVM.

Case 3: A 28-year-old woman was shot in the occipital area and rendered unconscious. She recovered consciousness many hours later. The bullet had not penetrated her skull. Some months later she began to see "rainbows" lasting for 2 to 5 minutes. Also, she seemed to experience some loss of vision. These symptoms, which were similar to migrainous phenomena, were not followed by headaches, although she had intermittent neuralgic occipital pain.

A few months later she had a generalized tonic-clonic seizure. EEG revealed occipital spikes. A CT scan was unremarkable. Initial treatment was with phenytoin. This failed to completely control her partial seizures, so carbamazepine was added. The two drugs in combination effectively controlled her seizures. One year later she was admitted to the hospital emergency department with continuous convulsions. Her phenytoin and carbamazepine concentrations were in the therapeutic range. Video-EEG showed no epileptiform activity during the seizures. Counseling for post-stress syndrome was instituted because it was clear that she was suffering from nonepileptic seizures of psychogenic origin. About 2 years after onset, she stopped having simple partial seizures, and the dose of phenytoin was gradually reduced, and then eliminated. Then her dose of carbamazepine was reduced to obtain levels of 4 to 6 µg/mL. Over time, her seizure threshold increased, that is, her propensity to have seizures decreased.

Seizure types: simple partial seizures with sensory symptoms (**I.** A.2); secondarily generalized tonic-clonic seizures (**I. C**); and nonepileptic seizures.

Epileptic syndrome: localization-related, symptomatic, and nonepileptic psychogenic (1.2)

Etiology: posttraumatic (for epileptic) and stress (for nonepileptic)

Prognosis: improvement over time

Case 4: A 7-year-old girl had a sudden decline in school performance. Her teacher noted frequent episodes of staring and blinking. A physician, suspicious of absence seizures, ordered an EEG. This was normal until she began hyperventilating, which induced an absence seizure with 3-per-second spike-and-wave discharges. She was treated with ethosuximide. Her school performance returned to its normal level. When she reached 12 years of age, the medication was tapered, and then discontinued. EEG was normal both during rest and hyperventilation.

Seizure type: absence (**II.** A)

Epileptic syndrome: childhood absence epilepsy (2.1)

Etiology: idiopathic

Prognosis: remission

References

1. Leppik IE: Epileptic syndromes: Genetic, diagnostic, and therapeutic aspects: introductory remarks and symposium overview. *Epilepsia* 1990;31(suppl 3):S1-S2.

2. Commission on Classification and Terminology of the International League Against Epilepsy: proposal for the classification of epilepsy and epileptic syndromes. *Epilepsia* 1989;30:389-399.

3. Delgado-Escueta AV, Treiman DM, Walsh GO: The treatable epilepsies. *N Engl J Med* 1983;308:1508-1514.

4. Peters HC, Kammer G, Volz A, et al: Mapping, genomic structure, and polymorphisms of the human GABABR1 receptor gene: evaluation of its involvement in idiopathic generalized epilepsy. *Neurogenetics* 1998;2(1):47-54.

5. Berkovic SF: Epilepsy genes and the genetics of epilepsy syndromes: the promise of new therapies based on genetic knowledge. *Epilepsia* 1997;38(suppl 9):S32-S36.

6. Cavazzutti GB: Epidemiology of different types of epilepsy in school-age children of Modena, Italy. *Epilepsia* 1980;21:57-62.

7. Loisseau P, Beaussart M: The benign seizures of childhood with rolandic paroxysmal discharges. *Epilepsia* 1973;14:381-389.

8. Bray PF, Wiser WC: Evidence for a genetic etiology of temporal-central abnormalities in focal epilepsy. *N Engl J Med* 1964;271:926-933.

9. Neubauer BA, Fiedler B, Himmelein B, et al: Centrotemporal spikes in families with rolandic epilepsy: linkage to chromosome 15q14. *Neurology* 1998;51(6):1608-1612.

10. Beaussart M, Faou R: Evolution of epilepsy with rolandic paroxysmal foci, a study of 324 cases. *Epilepsia* 1978;19:337.

11. Singh NA, Charlier C, Stauffer D, et al: A novel potassium channel gene, KCNQZ, is mutated in an inherited epilepsy of newborns. *Nat Genet* 1998;18:25-29.

12. Dreifuss FE: The epilepsies: clinical implications of the international classification. *Epilepsia* 1990;31(suppl 3):S3-S10.

13. Penry JK, Porter RJ, Dreifuss FE: Simultaneous recording of absence seizures with video tape and electroencephalography: a study of 374 seizures in 48 patients. *Brain* 1975;98:427-440.

14. Liu AW, Delgado-Escueto AV, Serratosa JM, et al: Juvenile myoclonic epilepsy locus in chromosome 6p21.2-p11: linkage to convulsions and electroencephalography trait. *Am J Hum Genet* 1995;57:368-381.

15. Kellaway P, Hrachovy RA, Frost JD, et al: Precise characterization and quantification of infantile spasms. *Ann Neurol* 1979;6:214-218.

16. Riikonen R, Donner M: ACTH therapy in infantile spasms, side effects. *Arch Dis Child* 1980;55:664-672.

17. Gastaut H, Roger J, Soulayrol R, et al: Childhood epileptic encephalopathy with diffuse slow spike-waves (otherwise known as "petit mal variant"). *Epilepsia* 1966;7:139-179.

18. Markland ON: Slow spike-wave activity in EEG and associated clinical features: often called Lennox or Lennox-Gastaut syndrome. *Neurology* 1977;27:746-757.

19. The Felbamate Study Group in Lennox-Gastaut syndrome. Efficacy of felbamate in childhood epileptic encephalopathy (Lennox-Gastaut syndrome). *N Engl J Med* 1993;328:29-33.

20. Nelson KB, Ellenberg JH: Predictors of epilepsy in children who have experienced febrile seizures. *N Engl J Med* 1976;295:1029-1033.

21. Wallace RH, Wang DW, Singh R, et al: Febrile seizures and generalized epilepsy associated with a mutation in the Na+-channel beta1 subunit gene SCN1B. *Nat Genet* 1998;19(4):366-370.

22. Nelson KB, Ellenberg JH: Prognosis in children with febrile seizures. *Pediatrics* 1978;61:720-727.

23. Nelson KB: Can treatment of febrile seizures prevent subsequent epilepsy? In: *Febrile Seizures*. Nelson KB, Ellenberg JH, eds. New York, Raven Press, 1981, pp 143-146.

24. Annegers JF, Hauser WA, Shirts SB, et al: Factors prognostic of unprovoked seizures after febrile convulsions. *N Engl J Med* 1987;316:493-498.

25. Fishman MA: Febrile seizures: the treatment controversy. *J Pediatr* 1979;94:177-184.

26. Farwell JR, Young JL, Hirtz DG, et al: Phenobarbital for febrile seizures: effects on intelligence and seizure recurrence. *N Engl J Med* 1990;322:364-369.

27. Augrell S, Berlin A, Ferngren H, et al: Plasma levels of diazepam after parenteral and rectal administration in children. *Epilepsia* 1975;16:277-283.

28. Kanto J: Plasma concentrations of diazepam and its metabolites after peroral, intramuscular and rectal administration. *Int J Clin Pharmacol* 1975;12:427-432.

29. Thorn I: Prevention of recurrent febrile seizures: intermittent prophylaxis with diazepam compared with continuous treatment with phenobarbital. In: *Febrile Seizures.* Nelson KB, Ellenberg JH, eds. New York, Raven Press, 1981, pp 119-126.

30. Dreifuss FE, Rosman NP, Cloyd JC, et al: A comparison of rectal diazepam gel and placebo for acute repetitive seizures. *N Engl J Med* 1998;338:1869-1875.

Chapter 4

Evaluation of a Seizure

T he most difficult step in evaluating a presumed seizure is determining if it was an epileptic seizure, or if it was a nonepileptic seizure or other event (Table 1). Most events associated with loss of consciousness and abnormal body movements are *not* epileptic seizures (as defined in Chapter 1). Events may be mistaken for seizures upon initial presentation, but must be differentiated from epileptic seizures because their treatment is different.

The second most difficult step when evaluating a presumed seizure is determining if the seizure portends the development of epilepsy. Not every seizure develops into epilepsy. The cumulative lifetime incidence rate for having at least one seizure is almost 9%, but the cumulative lifetime incidence of epilepsy is approximately 3%,[1] which means that only one third of persons who have a seizure ever develop epilepsy. Approximately one third of the 9% lifetime rate consists of children with uncomplicated febrile seizures who have no further seizures later in life and are not considered to have epilepsy. Another one third are persons who have only a single, isolated seizure, or have seizures in the context of a specific medical illness. The remaining one third of persons will develop recurrent seizures and be diagnosed as having epilepsy.

Thus, the occurrence of a seizure does not necessarily imply the presence of epilepsy. But a single seizure may be the

---

Table 1: Some Conditions That May Be Mistaken for Seizures

1. Syncope (see Table 4)
2. Nonepileptic seizures of psychogenic origin (pseudoseizures or psychogenic seizures)
3. Breath-holding spells
4. Paroxysmal REM sleep behavior
5. Panic attack

Table 2: Evaluation of a Single Seizure

History of the Event

1. Careful review of events occurring days before the seizure

2. Presence of any prodromal symptoms (auras)

3. Description of seizure and circumstantial evidence should be obtained from a reliable observer and witness

4. Postictal observations—time to recovery of normal function and any neurologic deficits

Medical History

1. Febrile convulsions

2. Head injury

3. Cerebrovascular or cardiovascular disease

4. Cancer

5. Substance abuse

6. Infectious disease

Family History

1. Febrile convulsions

2. Epilepsy in siblings, parents, or close relatives

3. History of neurologic disorders

Social History

1. Travel

2. Occupation

Physical Examination

1. Injury pattern

2. Cardiovascular system

3. Skin

Neurologic Examination

1. Focal postictal deficits

2. Focal neurologic deficits after recovery

3. Neuropsychologic assessment

Laboratory Evaluation

1. EEG

2. Structural study, MRI preferable

3. Routine laboratory assessment

4. Toxicologic screen

Table 3: Differential Diagnosis of Syncope

1. Vasovagal attack
   - hyperventilation-induced syncope
2. Cardiac
   - atrioventricular block
   - Adams-Stokes attack
   - sinoatrial block
   - paroxysmal tachycardia
   - reflex cardiac arrhythmia
   - other cardiac causes of decreased cardiac output
3. Hypovolemia
4. Hypotension
5. Cerebrovascular ischemia
6. Micturition syncope

initial event heralding epilepsy. To make an accurate determination about the probability of further seizures, a detailed evaluation must be performed (Table 2).

Syncope and Other Conditions

One of the physician's most important tasks in evaluating a patient with an episode of loss of consciousness is to determine if the event was a seizure or syncope.[2] Syncopal events are the most common symptoms confused with seizures, especially if there is inadequate history or observational data. There are many causes of syncope (Table 3). Brief clonic activity often accompanies syncope, and this can often lead to confusion regarding the diagnosis. However, the character of the muscle activity in syncope is mostly clonic or myoclonic, involves distal extremities, and rarely causes the classical axial tonic posturing seen in a tonic-clonic seizure. For example, a medical student, after donating blood and suffering from sleep deprivation, stood up, became pale, lost consciousness, fell slowly to the ground, exhibited some clonic activity of his hands, and lost bladder sphincter control. Although he was initially diagnosed as having had a seizure, the setting of the event and clinical features later led to the more accurate diagnosis of syncope. Table 4 lists those features that may help in differentiating syncope from seizures.

Table 4: Clinical Features and Diagnostic Tests to Help Differentiate Generalized Tonic-Clonic Seizures and Syncope

Clinical finding	Seizure	Syncope
Injury*	common	rare
Urinary incontinence	common	rare
Confusion after event	common	rare
Headache	common	rare
Focal neurological findings	sometimes	never
Related to posture	no	often
Skin color	cyanotic	pale
Premonitory symptoms	short	long
Diagnostic tests		
Prolactin level	elevated	normal
Abnormal EEG	common	rare
Abnormal ECG	rare	sometimes

*The pattern of injury may be very helpful. Tongue or cheek biting is common with convulsions, rare with syncope. Some malingerers will bite the tip of the tongue, whereas with convulsions, usually only one side of the tongue is bitten by the molars. Persons with convulsions often fall forward or backward while the body is tonic or rigid, thus injuring the forehead, chin, or occipital area. Persons with syncope generally have gentler falls than persons with seizures.

Cardiogenic syncope is seen most often in the elderly (Table 3). Micturition syncope and cough syncope[3,4] are reflex events leading to hypotension, loss of consciousness, falls, and sometimes injury. Cardiac causes of syncope must be considered, and can often be diagnosed by electrocardiogram (ECG).[5,6]

The terms psychogenic or pseudoseizure are being replaced by the more specific and less pejorative term, nonepileptic (NEE) seizure of psychogenic origin. These events are often dramatic, with much motor activity that is usually considerably more complex than simple tonic-clonic activity. There may be pelvic thrusting, side-to-side head shaking, asynchronous extremity movements, and other embellishments. Patients with these seizures, if properly diagnosed and treated, can have a favorable outcome.[7] Unfortunately, frontal lobe seizures may also present as unusual and violent motor behaviors with minimal EEG findings. The differential diagnosis between nonepileptic and frontal lobe seizures may be difficult.

In the past, breath-holding spells in children were considered to be possible seizures. But they have clearly been shown to be nonepileptic and associated with behavioral problems. They may be associated with cyanosis or pallor.[8]

History of the Event

Most seizures occur in the absence of trained observers. Moreover, many persons who witness a seizure for the first time are often too frightened or preoccupied with trying to help the stricken person to observe events carefully. It would be useful to know if a seizure began as a partial seizure that then generalized, or if it was generalized from the onset. But this determination about how a seizure originated is rarely based on first-hand observation. Most of the seizures that attract attention are generalized tonic-clonic seizures. Yet, most adults have localization-related epilepsy with partial seizures. Often, partial seizures are not recognized as significant events, and they may be present for some time before a secondarily generalized seizure occurs. For example, for months one of my patients had episodes of staring at the television and not responding to his wife before he eventually had a generalized tonic-clonic seizure that led to his hospital admission. Structural studies revealed a glioma, and, in retrospect, the staring spells were complex partial seizures.

Events occurring before the seizure must be reviewed. It is important to determine if the seizure was provoked or unprovoked. Unprovoked means that there was no specific disturbance of homeostasis and that the event was truly paroxysmal. Many things can provoke seizures. A common example is college students who experience seizures after extensive sleep deprivation and excessive use of stimulants when preparing for examinations. The most frequent examples of provoked seizures are febrile convulsions that occur only during a high fever. Provoked seizures are much less likely to be predictive of subsequent epilepsy. Table 5 is a list of events that

Table 5: Some Common Causes of Provoked Seizures

1. Massive sleep deprivation
2. Excessive use of stimulants
3. Withdrawal from sedative drugs or alcohol
4. Substance abuse (cocaine, methamphetamine)
5. High fever
6. Hypoglycemia
7. Electrolyte imbalance
8. Hypoxia

may precipitate seizures but do not have a high association with the development of epilepsy.

Sometimes a patient, after fully recovering from the effect of the seizure, will recall prodromal symptoms. For example, the patient evaluated in case report 3 of Chapter 3 did not discuss the visual symptoms of seeing rainbows until after she had fully recovered from her generalized tonic-clonic seizure, and then only after she was asked if she had any unusual visual phenomena. The information pointing to focal neurologic involvement can be crucial in helping classify and, more importantly, localize, the onset of a seizure.

Medical History

A careful review of a patient's medical history is necessary. This may be impossible during or immediately after the seizure because the patient may be postictal, confused, disoriented, or unable or unwilling to disclose sensitive information, such as drug abuse. For example, a woman from the Twin Cities went to Arizona to visit relatives. A few days after arriving, she had two generalized tonic-clonic seizures in one day. She was told she had epilepsy and was started on antiepileptic medications. Upon returning, she was reevaluated, and only after a thorough review of events surrounding the seizure did she reveal that she had been a heavy user of benzodiazepines for sleep and anxiety, and had forgotten to take her medications to Arizona. In retrospect, she had seizures provoked by benzodiazepine withdrawal.

Because their parents never tell them, many persons do not know that they had febrile convulsions as children. Many families regard epilepsy as an embarrassment and often never reveal to the rest of the family the fact that a relative has had the disorder. Obviously, travel, work stress, sleep deprivation, and other factors may be important and must be fully evaluated.

Physical Examination

The first physician to evaluate the patient must perform a careful physical examination, directed toward finding specific signs that would help determine if the event was a seizure, and, if so, establishing its cause.

During a generalized tonic-clonic seizure, the CNS is in a state of maximal excitation, and all systems influenced by the brain are in a state of stimulation. Pulse rate increases, blood pressure rises, salivation increases, pupils dilate, and there is an excessive release of some hormones, such as prolactin. Respirations cease in the tonic phase and may be irregular in the clonic phase. The patient may appear frighteningly cyanotic in the tonic phase, but this color may be misleading because during the tonic phase intrathoracic pressure is increased and venous return is impeded, resulting in increased volume of desaturated blood in the face. After the seizure, there is respiratory and metabolic acidosis, and the response to this is marked increase in respiratory drive. Objects should not be placed in the patient's mouth because these may impede respiration and induce vomiting.

Vital Signs

After generalized tonic-clonic seizures, the pulse is usually strong and rapid. Depending on the patient's physical condition and age, tachycardia may persist for a few minutes or much longer. One of my patients once compared the physical exertion of a tonic-clonic seizure to running 1 mile. Although the seizure is usually only 1 or 2 minutes long, all major muscle groups are maximally contracted. This places considerable stress on the cardiovascular system, which is usually well tolerated by younger patients but may cause problems in the elderly. The presence of cardiac arrhythmias suggests that the seizure may have been related to a cardiogenic event resulting in cerebral hypoxia.

Respirations after a generalized tonic-clonic seizure are usually deep and rapid as the patient hyperventilates to overcome the respiratory acidosis, lactacidemia, and oxygen depletion. After syncope, respirations are usually normal. Patients who have had hyperventilation-induced syncope often experience apnea or have a slowed respiratory rate because of the hypocarbia. Airway patency must be evaluated. For example, a Minnesota Twins fan was treated for what were initially thought to be epileptic seizures during an exciting game. But it was quickly determined that his condition was the result of an aspirated hot dog leading to cerebral hypoxia.

Blood pressure is usually elevated for a few minutes after a generalized tonic-clonic seizure. Hypotension is unusual after a seizure, but its presence in the elderly may suggest the occurrence of a myocardial infarction.

After a single, generalized tonic-clonic seizure, body temperature is usually normal. The presence of fever raises the possibility of a reactive seizure, such as a benign febrile convulsion in children or an infection in adults.

General Appearance

Most patients are comatose, lethargic, or confused after a generalized tonic-clonic seizure. Hyperexcitability, aggression, or agitation are unusual and may suggest the patient's use of drugs or a psychological disorder.

HEENT

Examination of the head can be very informative. First, signs of new and old trauma must be assessed because injuries are common with a tonic-clonic seizure. The body becomes rigid, the patient loses consciousness, and falls either forward or backward, depending on the posture of the body at the onset of the seizure. With syncope, there is usually a prolonged prodromal period and the patient usually "slides" to the ground because consciousness is not abruptly lost. Scars can be important clues to past head injuries and intracranial surgery that may predispose a patient to seizures and epilepsy. Because patients with severe, intractable epilepsy have frequent falls either forward or backward, multiple scars with thickening of subcutaneous tissue develop on the chin, forehead, and occipital area. Injuries to the side of the head are much less common from seizures.

Tongue biting is a common consequence of a tonic-clonic seizure. Usually, one side of the tongue is bitten with the molars or incisors as the tongue is trapped by the tonic contraction of the masseter muscles. Occasionally, patients with nonepileptic seizures, knowing the importance of tongue biting, will intentionally bite the tip of their tongue to give the appearance of a seizure. These bites, however, are usually very shallow and do not bleed as profusely as the involuntary tongue bites with an epileptic seizure.

Teeth fractures may occur from falls associated with generalized tonic-clonic seizures, but are rare in other kinds of seizures.

Excessive salivation occurs from stimulation of the parotid glands and from tonic contraction of the masseter muscles that empty the contents into the oral cavity. This, coupled with rapid, deep respiration after the seizure, leads to the classical frothing at the mouth. This is not usually seen in patients with nonepileptic seizures but cases of malingerers using soap to imitate the frothing have been reported throughout history.[9]

Clear fluid that drains from the nose may indicate the leakage of cerebrospinal fluid from a fracture of the cribriform plate resulting from a skull fracture.

An asymmetrical head may be a clue to the presence of underlying injury to the brain in early childhood.

Careful examination of the eyes may reveal small neurofibromatoses of the iris as a clue to the presence of von Recklinghausen's disease. Funduscopic examination may show papilledema, a sign of increased intracranial pressure from tumor, pseudotumor cerebri, or recent intracerebral hemorrhage. The presence of optic atrophy, macular degeneration, "cherry red spot/mulberry" tumor (tuberous sclerosis), angiomatosis retinae of von Hippel-Lindau disease, and other anomalies open specific areas for differential diagnosis and need further evaluation.

A patient's dysmorphic facial features should be evaluated because they may provide clues to specific syndromes. For example, patients with Down syndrome may develop epilepsy in adulthood.

Neck

The neck must be examined for injuries. Fracture of the cervical spine may occur during a seizure-precipitated fall.

Hyperthyroidism or parahyperthyroidism may be associated with seizures. Presence of carotid bruits should direct attention to cerebrovascular causes of seizures.

Lungs

Aspiration may occur in the postictal state, especially if vomiting has been induced by attempts to place tongue blades or other objects into the mouth. Pneumonia and other respiratory illness may be accompanied by febrile seizures.

Heart

A thorough search should be made for cardiac disorders. It is not unusual to find patients treated for epilepsy who have a cardiac condition leading to cerebral hypoxia. In young adults, conduction defects may be present but overlooked. In the elderly, Adams-Stokes syndrome attacks, cardiac arrhythmias, and other conditions may be the etiologic factors (Table 3). The presence of a new myocardial infarction from the stress of a seizure must be excluded in the elderly patient.

Genitourinary

Loss of urine has been the hallmark of an epileptic attack since antiquity.[10] The Greeks knew that the loss of urine occurred after the tonic-clonic seizure. In fact, they considered the loss of urine and feces the seizure's terminal event, the body's expelling of the evil humors that were thought to cause the epilepsy. The release of urine is caused by relaxation of the sphincters in the postictal state and depends on the depth of coma after the seizure. In a patient with treated epilepsy, seizures are often less severe and not associated with loss of bowel or bladder sphincter tone. Thus, the absence of incontinence does not exclude the event from having been a seizure. Conversely, the presence of urinary incontinence does not establish the presence of a seizure. Some patients with profound syncope will experience incontinence, and some malingerers will deliberately soil themselves.

Extremities

Fractures and soft-tissue injuries may occur as a consequence of generalized tonic-clonic seizures. Burns may be seen in patients with complex partial seizures. Injuries are much less common from vasovagal syncope.

Table 6: The Neurocutaneous Syndromes (Phakomatoses)

All of these are characteristic syndromes with specific findings and are noted primarily for their tendency to be expressed in the skin and brain, although other organs may be involved. All but Sturge-Weber syndrome are inherited.

- Neurofibromatosis (von Recklinghausen's disease)
- Tuberous sclerosis
- von Hippel-Lindau disease
- Ataxia-telangiectasia (Louis-Bar's syndrome)
- Sturge-Weber syndrome (encephalofacial angiomatosis)

Unilateral smallness of hands and feet is seen in patients who have had early childhood brain injuries or intrauterine injuries. These may be unrecognized for many years and present as signs of epilepsy only later.

Skin

A number of neurocutaneous syndromes (phakomatoses, from the Greek "phakos," meaning birth mark) have specific manifestations (Table 6).[11] Neurofibromatosis is an autosomal-dominant disorder with variable clinical expression and occurs in 1 of 4,000 persons. The diagnostic criteria are six or more café au lait spots, two or more neurofibromas, and/or various combinations of bone dysplasias, optic glioma, or having a first-degree relative with the diagnosis. In tuberous sclerosis, the characteristic lesions are adenoma sebaceum (which should not be confused with acne) and hypopigmented skin areas. It is an autosomal-dominant condition affecting 1 in 30,000. Sturge-Weber syndrome consists of a facial nevus (port-wine stain) of the upper face often associated with ipsilateral intracranial calcifications. The cutaneous telangiectasia in Louis-Bar's syndrome may be difficult to spot but are most common on exposed areas of skin.

Neurologic Examination

Mental Status. After the seizure, the postictal period (from the Greek "ictus," to seize) is an important time to search for clues that would help determine if the event was a seizure or another problem. Time to recovery of normal function is important (Table 4). Patients with syncope or nonepileptic seizures are usually lucid immediately after or within a few minutes of the event. Patients may be obviously confused for some time after a tonic-clonic seizure and, if carefully tested, found to have significant memory impairment for many hours and sometimes days. They may also have considerable retrograde amnesia for the event. One of my patients had been on a stressful trip, lost sleep, used alcohol, lost consciousness on his drive from the airport, and drove his car into a tree near his home. No one witnessed the event, but because he had lost bladder and bowel control, had bitten his tongue, and had been unconscious and far more confused than what would have been expected for this kind of accident, we concluded that he had had a provoked seizure.

Speech difficulties such as aphasia or anomia can be important clues to the lateralization of the onset of seizures. However, a patient's difficulty in speaking because of confusion or lingual injury from the seizure must be considered in the evaluation.

Cranial Nerves. Absence of the sense of smell may be caused by a fracture of the cribriform plate from recent or old head trauma.

Visual-field defect may be a prominent finding after a seizure if it had its onset in the occipital lobe. This can be of important lateralization value. The patient in case report 3 of Chapter 3 would often have an easily detectable scotoma (area of visual loss) for some hours after her seizure.

Asymmetrical pupils, especially a large unreactive one, suggest the presence of uncal herniation from a large intra-cranial mass such as an epidural hematoma and require immediate evaluation. Small unreactive pupils may be associated with drug abuse.

Facial asymmetry may signify the presence of a stroke or, rarely, may be postictal.

Motor. Presence of postictal Todd's paralysis can be an important clue to help localize the brain region from which the seizure emanated. Weakness of one hand, for example, will point to the contralateral motor area. This information needs to be communicated to the radiologist so that specific views of the areas in question can be obtained.

Sensory. Unilateral sensory loss suggests an intracranial lesion in the contralateral parietal lobe.

Reflexes. Asymmetry of reflexes can be a useful clue to the hemisphere of origin of a seizure. The presence of a pathological reflex, such as Babinski's sign, may persist for hours after a seizure.

Laboratory Evaluation

Appropriate laboratory testing is essential in supplementing the patient's history and physical examination. The major tests are sampling of bodily fluids (blood, cerebrospinal fluid), imaging studies (MRI), neurophysiologic studies (electroencephalogram), and functional tests (IQ testing, behavioral testing). Different sets of tests are needed, depending on the phase of the disorder. Acute evaluations are done as soon as possible after the initial seizure or onset of epilepsy; if the seizures develop into intractable epilepsy, more sophisticated evaluation is necessary to fully treat the patient for seizure control and for integration into society.

Blood

Glucose levels should be measured routinely in patients presenting to the emergency room with seizures of undetermined origin. In patients with epilepsy, blood glucose concentrations do not decrease significantly after generalized tonic-clonic seizures. However, both hypoglycemia and hyperglycemia can cause seizures.

In adults, blood glucose concentrations of less than 40 mg/dL may precipitate seizures. Seizures associated with hypoglycemia usually have a prodromal period characterized by weakness, confusion, and other symptoms, and the tonic-clonic phase may be associated with less vigorous motor activity. Treatment with antiepileptic medication is ineffective, and not recognizing and treating the hypoglycemia may lead to CNS damage.

Nonketotic hyperosmotic hyperglycemia may be characterized by both partial and generalized seizures. In these patients, blood glucose values of greater than 350 mg/dL are observed. Again, treatment of the underlying metabolic disturbance is essential. However, some patients with diabetes develop epilepsy from a lesion in the CNS. Poor control of diabetes may be associated with increased seizures, even without the extremes of blood glucose levels needed for hypoglycemic or hyperglycemic seizures. Phenytoin may affect release of insulin from the pancreas and thus may modify insulin requirements. The glucose tolerance test may be affected by phenytoin use.

In patients with epilepsy, carbamazepine may induce mild to moderate hyponatremia with sodium levels of 130 mEq/L. Most patients with mild hyponatremia associated with use of carbamazepine are not symptomatic, and the low sodium levels can be treated by water restriction. Severe hyponatremia, hypomagnesemia, and other electrolyte imbalances may cause seizures, but this is usually seen in the context of other illnesses.

Alcohol abuse is often associated with seizures. Usually, the seizures occur within 48 hours of the last drink and may be the brain's response to the withdrawal from alcohol. Blood alcohol levels may be low at the time of the seizure. A first seizure, even in the presence of alcohol use, should be fully evaluated, however, because sometimes the alcohol use triggers a seizure from CNS pathology. Also, some patients who abuse alcohol and have withdrawal seizures may eventually develop epilepsy, possibly from recurrent head trauma.

Drug abuse is another common cause of seizures, either from acute use or from withdrawal. Most drugs that are CNS stimulants can cause acute seizures. These include cocaine, amphetamines, PCP, and others. Measurable concentrations of these drugs may be found in blood or urine at the time of the seizure. Most sedative drugs such as barbiturates or benzodiazepines cause seizures only after withdrawal from chronic use, and measurable amounts of these may not be present in biological fluids at the time of the seizure.

An interesting finding is that prolactin is elevated after epileptic seizures but not after nonepileptic psychogenic seizures.[12] The rise is usually dramatic, with levels increasing two to four times over baseline levels. However, the levels might not rise after partial seizures, and they may already be high from treatment with psychotropic drugs. Nevertheless, when one suspects nonepileptic seizures, a prolactin level should be obtained 15 to 30 minutes after the seizure.

A lumbar puncture should be done whenever CNS infection is suspected. However, after serial seizures, there may be a few white cells in the spinal fluid, findings that may be confused with viral infections of the CNS. The minor pleocytosis from seizures is usually not enough to be confused with bacterial meningitis, which is accompanied by a few hundred or more white cells. Tubercular meningitis usually has elevated protein. Herpes encephalitis usually is accompanied by both white and red blood cells.

The most common cause of blood in the cerebrospinal fluid (CSF) is head trauma. In such injuries, microscopic examination reveals red blood cell (RBC) counts of 100 to several thousand per cubic mm. On the other hand, after subarachnoid hemorrhage, the CSF is grossly bloody, and the RBC count often exceeds $100,000/mm^3$.

EEG

The electroencephalogram (EEG) is as vital to the diagnosis of seizures as is the ECG to cardiac disorders. The EEG was developed in the early part of this century and has played an important role in our understanding of epilepsy. One of its first successes was in identifying the classical 3-per-second spike-and-wave pattern characteristic of absence ("petit mal") seizure. Subsequent use of the EEG has confirmed its utility as a tool for diagnosing and classifying the epilepsies.

The background rhythm of a normal waking EEG consists of alpha activity of 20 to 50 µV (20 to 50 millionths of a volt). This activity is less than one hundreth of the amplitude of cardiac potentials. Thus, the EEG signals are much more difficult to detect, and with DC amplifiers, the EEG signals would be completely masked by muscle and cardiac activity. However, the development of AC amplifiers and bipolar recording has made it possible to measure the small, brain-generated potentials. But it should be obvious that in the presence of many relatively higher physiologic potentials, the EEG is subject to a great deal of artifact. Indeed, the most difficult aspect of EEG interpretation is correctly recognizing artifacts and not misinterpreting them as pathological. Many mistakes have been made in diagnosing the presence of epilepsy when the abnormality later was determined to be artifact. Guidelines have been established for the proper technical qualifi-

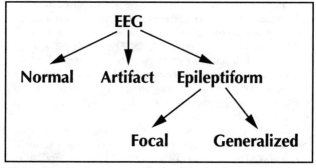

Figure 1—*EEG findings and the differential diagnosis of seizures. When the EEG contains epileptiform activity, the clinical diagnosis of epilepsy is secure and can be classified as localization-related (focal) or generalized. A normal EEG does not exclude the diagnosis of epilepsy. Artifact is troubling because it may be misinterpreted as epileptic, leading to an incorrect clinical diagnosis.*

cations for EEG laboratories and technicians, as have specialty boards for electroencephalographers.

An EEG requires the placement of 21 standard electrodes over the scalp. Additional electrodes, such as sphenoidal or nasopharyngeal, may be used in some laboratories if there is a question of complex partial seizures.[13] Care must be taken to apply electrodes properly, because movement of the contacts can generate potentials that may be much larger than the underlying EEG potentials. Also, because ECG artifact may be recorded easily, the use of a special channel to monitor the ECG is advisable so that these potentials can be recognized as cardiac in origin.

The EEG electrodes are connected to the amplifiers in pairs. These can be linked up into montages in a number of ways, and although there are general guides, many laboratories have developed their own specific configurations. Most modern EEG machines have 16 channels. These are recorded simultaneously because it is necessary to be able to develop a "map" of abnormal activity. In addition, since seizures may in some instances be triggered by hyperventilation or photic

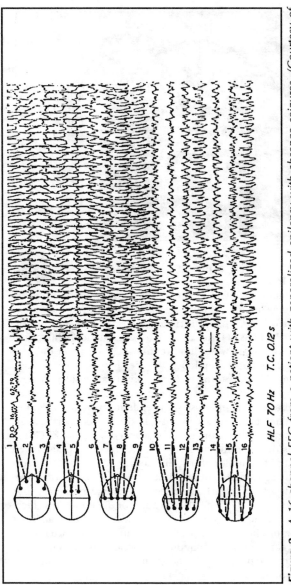

Figure 2—A 16-channel EEG from a patient with generalized epilepsy with absence seizures. (Courtesy of Fernando Torres, MD).

HLF 70 Hz   T.C. 0.12 s

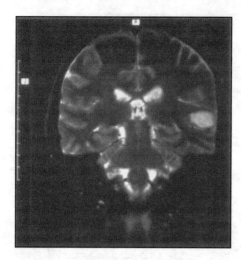

Figure 3—An MRI scan from a patient diagnosed with complex partial seizures from a glioma. A CT scan had been normal.

stimulation, these activation techniques should be performed in all EEGs.[13]

A major problem in the diagnosis of epilepsy is that the EEG may be normal for long periods relative to the time of the recording. Epileptiform activity is present only at brief intervals. Thus, it is not uncommon for a standard 30-minute recording to show no definite interictal activity in the presence of diagnosed epilepsy. Studies have shown that only 50% to 60% of routine EEGs (30 minutes, no sleep deprivation) obtained after a seizure in patients later clearly diagnosed as having epilepsy show epileptiform abnormalities. While normal EEGs are not useful, abnormal recordings are very helpful. Two things can be learned from the EEG. The first is the determination of the presence of epilepsy. The finding of an epileptiform EEG and the history of a seizure are strong evidence of the existence of a CNS disorder associated with a risk for further seizures. The second major purpose of the EEG is the classification of the epilepsy as localization-related or generalized. In addition, the localization of the discharge is helpful in determining the area of the brain containing the epileptogenic lesion (Figure 1). Knowledge of the probable site of origin can help guide other diagnostic studies.

The signature of an epileptic EEG abnormality is the sharp transient, which is usually a spike (less than 80 milliseconds) or a sharp wave (longer than a spike). A number of computer programs have been developed for spike detection, but for clinical diagnosis visual interpretation is still needed to screen out artifacts and place the occurrence of these sharp transients into clinical perspective. Spikes may be focal or generalized. Focal spikes are most often seen in the temporal regions. Muscle artifact, ECG potential, movement artifacts, and "electrode pops" must be differentiated from activity of CNS origin.

One of the most common errors made is the misreading of ECG potential or other sharp activity as spikes. In the intensive care unit, even the electromagnetic field generated by a drop of saline may be recorded and appear as a spike. In addition, there are cerebral potentials such as small sharp spikes, 14 and 6 spike and wave complexes, and other phenomena that have been misinterpreted as abnormal but now have been clearly established to be variants of normal activity occurring in some patients.[14] An example of EEG activity is shown in Figure 2.

CT and MRI

Structural studies should be done in localization-related epilepsy, especially if the history and clinical findings suggest the possibility of an intra-cranial lesion. In the past, CT scans were the diagnostic study of choice, but the MRI is now much more useful because of its better resolution. The CT scan is acceptable for determining the existence of vascular lesions and certain tumors larger than 1 cm, as well as regions of brain injury. However, low-grade gliomas that may be isodense with surrounding brain or subtle atrophy, especially in the temporal regions, are missed with the CT scan (Figure 3). In addition, MRIs are now able to detect subtle congenital malformations, such as cortical heterotopias.

Patients with mesial temporal sclerosis, who constitute a large fraction of patients with intractable epilepsy, may now be diagnosed by MRI. These "scars" of the mesial temporal lobe are rarely detected by CT scans. Yet, the detection of unilateral mesial temporal sclerosis by MRI is valuable information when evaluating a patient for surgery. In one review of seven reports in the literature, evaluating a total of 341 patients with epilepsy who had both CT and MRI scans, the MRI was superior in almost all of them. The overall detection rate of abnormalities was 32% for CT and 42% for MRI.[15]

References

1. Hauser WA, Kurland LT: The epidemiology of epilepsy in Rochester, Minnesota, 1935 through 1967. *Epilepsia* 1975;16:1-66.

2. Kapoor WN, Karpf M, Wieaned S, et al: A prospective evaluation and follow-up of patients with syncope. *N Engl J Med* 1983;309:197-204.

3. Kerr A Jr, Derbes VJ: The syndrome of cough syncope. *Ann Intern Med* 1953;39:1240-1253.

4. DeMaria AA, Westmoreland BF, Sharbrough FW: EEG in cough syncope. *Neurology* 1984;34:371-374.

5. Peretz DI, Abdulla A: Management of cardioinhibitory hypersensitive carotid sinus syndrome with permanent cardiac pacing: a 17-year prospective study. *Can J Cardiol* 1985;1:86-91.

6. Schwartz PJ, Periti M, Malliani A: Long QT syndrome. *Am Heart J* 1975;89:378-390.

7. Ramani SV, Quesney LF, Olson D: Diagnosis of hysterical seizures in epileptic patients. *Am J Psychiatry* 1980;137:705-709.

8. Lombrosco CT, Lerman P: Breath-holding spells (cyanotic and pallid infantile syncope). *Pediatrics* 1967;39:563-581.

9. Temkin O: *The Falling Sickness: A History of Epilepsy from the Greeks to the Beginnings of Modern Neurology.* 2nd ed, revised. Baltimore and London, Johns Hopkins Press, 1971, p 166.

10. Temkin O: *The Falling Sickness: A History of Epilepsy from the Greeks to the Beginnings of Modern Neurology.* 2nd ed, revised. Baltimore and London, Johns Hopkins Press, 1971, p 327.

11. Berg BO: Neurocutaneous syndromes: phakomatoses and allied conditions. In: *Pediatric Neurology.* Vol 2. Swaiman KF, ed. St Louis, CV Mosby Co, 1989, pp 795-817.

12. Trimble MR: Serum prolactin in epilepsy and hysteria. *Br Med J* 1978;2:1682.

13. Aminoff MJ: Electroencephalography: General principles and clinical applications. In: Aminoff MJ, ed. *Electrodiagnosis in Clinical Neurology.* 2nd ed. New York, Churchill Livingstone, 1986, pp 21-77.

14. White JC, Langston JW, Pedley TA: Benign epileptiform transients of sleep. *Neurology* 1977;27:1061.

15. Riela AR, Penry JK: Magnetic resonance imaging. In: *Comprehensive Epileptology.* Dam M, Gram L, eds. New York, Raven Press, 1990, p 359.

Chapter 5

When to Start and When to Stop Treatment for Seizures

One of the most difficult decisions facing a physician caring for a patient with a seizure is deciding when to start treatment. This decision can be made only after the patient and his or her physician discuss and evaluate a number of issues. The first step is to assess the risk of further seizures.

If the seizures are nonepileptic, treatment must be directed at the underlying cause. Thus, hypoglycemic seizures of the neonate are treated with glucose, alcohol withdrawal seizures can best be controlled by altering addictive behavior, and seizures of psychogenic origin can be modified by appropriate counseling. Treatment of epileptic seizures is governed by assessing the risk of treatment against the benefit of using medications. One of the major reasons for being familiar with epilepsy syndromes is that knowledge of their natural history permits better identification of the risk of further seizures. For example, children with benign epilepsy with centrotemporal spikes may not need treatment with medications because studies have shown that they often outgrow this condition after experiencing only a few nocturnal seizures. Therefore, the overall risk of medication treatment may not be warranted.

Some structural lesions are clearly associated with recurrent seizures. These include brain tumor and arteriovenous malformation. When these are diagnosed after a single seizure, there should be no hesitation in initiating pharmacologic treatment and considering surgical resection. However, a much more common situation is the one in which the initial evaluation fails to reveal a specific provoking factor. Data from clinical studies in the last decade have identified specific risk factors, based on a complete evaluation, that help identify patients who are at higher risk for having additional seizures. The risk of a third seizure in a person who has had two unprovoked seizures is 73%.[1]

Table 1: When to Use Chronic Treatment With Antiepileptic Medication After a Single Seizure

If a single seizure is followed rapidly by a second seizure—for example, within the first day—treatment should be started regardless of etiology. An MRI, EEG, and careful examination are needed to make these decisions.

Definitely:

With structural lesion:

- Brain tumor, such as meningioma, glioma, neoplastic
- Arteriovenous malformation
- Infection, such as abscess, herpes encephalitis

Without structural lesion:

- History of epilepsy in sibling (but not parents)
- EEG with definite epileptic pattern
- History of prior acute seizure—a seizure in the context of an illness or a childhood febrile seizure
- History of brain injury or stroke, CNS infection, significant head trauma
- Todd's postictal paresis
- Status epilepticus at onset

Possibly:

- Unprovoked seizure with none of the above risk factors

Probably Not
(although short-term therapy may be used):

- Alcohol withdrawal
- Drug abuse
- Seizure in context of acute illness, ie, high fever, dehydration, hypoglycemia
- Postimpact seizure (a single seizure immediately after an acute blow to the head)
- A specific benign epilepsy syndrome such as febrile convulsions or benign epilepsy with centrotemporal spikes
- Seizure provoked by excessive sleep deprivation (eg, college student at examination time)

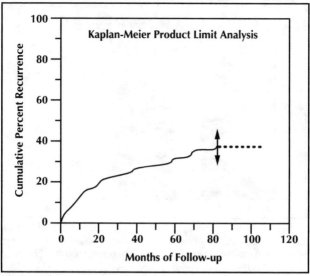

Figure 1—*Recurrence of seizures among 208 patients after a first unprovoked seizure. Arrows identify standard errors. Used with permission,* Neurology *1990.[2]*

Categories for Treatment

The decision to treat can be divided into three general categories: treat; possibly treat; and probably not treat, summarized in Table 1. The clinical research supporting these decisions has been developed in a series of papers for adults[2-8] and for children.[9-11]

Studies have found a recurrence rate of 34% to 71% after a single seizure in adults.[2,3] Variance among these studies can be explained in part by differences in study design, characteristics of populations, and duration of follow-up. Generally, the longer the follow-up, the higher the rate of recurrence.

A study of 208 patients, all of whom had one unprovoked seizure and were followed for more than 4 years (total of 853 patient years), found an overall risk of 34% for a second seizure at the end of 5 years[2] (Figure 1). Patients for this study (teenagers and adults) were drawn from hospital admissions

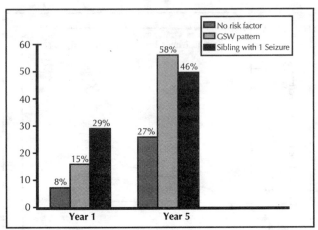

Figure 2—*The probability of a second seizure 1 and 5 years after a single seizure, based on three sets of factors: no known risk, a generalized spike-wave (GSW) pattern on the EEG, and a sibling with one or more seizures.*[2]

and referrals to EEG laboratories and neurology and epilepsy clinics at four hospitals (one university hospital, one Veterans Administration hospital, and two urban hospitals).

In this study, patients who had no history of a central nervous system (CNS) insult (idiopathic single seizure) had a recurrence risk of 10% at 1 year, 24% at 2 years, and 29% at 5 years. This group was evaluated for further risk factors. Family history was important. Among those with a single unprovoked seizure and a sibling with seizures, the recurrence rate was 29% at 1 year and 46% at 5 years, compared to 9% at 1 year and 26% at 5 years for those with no sibling with epilepsy (Figure 2). However, a history of seizures in parents or in first-degree relatives was not associated with a higher risk.

Another important predictive factor was the EEG. Patients with a pattern of generalized spikes and waves (GSW) had a recurrence risk of 15% at 1 year and 58% at 5 years, compared to 9% and 26%, respectively, for those with normal EEG or nonspecific EEG pattern (Figure 2).

Another important factor was the occurrence of a previous seizure in the context of an illness, or a childhood febrile

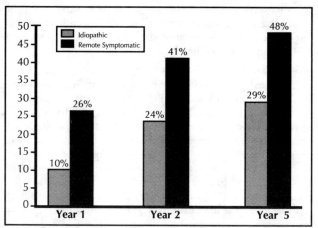

Figure 3—Recurrence risk for idiopathic (no known central nervous system injury) or remote symptomatic (previous stroke, head injury, infection, etc).[2]

seizure. These patients had a risk of 10% at 1 year and 39% at 5 years.

Age, gender, seizure type, abnormal EEG other than GSW, and abnormal neurologic examination did not elevate the risk above others in the idiopathic group.

Another group was categorized as "remote symptomatic." These were patients who had a history of head trauma, stroke, CNS infection, or static encephalopathy from birth with mental retardation or cerebral palsy. These patients had a risk for a second seizure of 26% at 1 year, 41% at 2 years, and 48% at 5 years, markedly higher than rates of 10%, 24%, and 29%, respectively, in those with no history of CNS damage (Figure 3).

Within the remote symptomatic group, increased risk for recurrence was found in those with Todd's postictal paresis—41% at 1 year and 75% at 5 years. If a prior acute seizure was present, the risk for a second seizure was 60% at 1 year and 80% at 5 years. If status epilepticus or multiple seizures occurred at onset, the recurrence rate was 37% at 1 year and 56% at 3 years.

Thus, a patient with a previous CNS insult, or with a sibling with seizures, or with prior acute seizure, or with a GSW-

EEG pattern, or with Todd's postictal paresis, has a significantly higher risk of a second seizure than a patient without these risk factors. Most neurologists would treat these patients with antiepileptic medications.

When Risk Factors Are Lacking

A more difficult decision arises for those patients with none of the additional risk factors. For these patients, the probability of a second seizure is less than 10% in the first year and approximately 24% by the end of 2 years after the single seizure. Is this a high enough rate to warrant the risks of treatment? There is no single answer to this question. The decision to treat or not to treat must be based on an evaluation by the patient and physician of the perceived risk and benefit. As described in other sections, the risk of treatment with available antiepileptic medications is generally low. The impact of a second seizure depends on the patient's life-style. Treatment may be indicated for patients needing to drive, or for those who face significant risk of injury or loss of self-esteem from a second seizure. The risk of recurrence is greatest in the first 2 years, so if treatment is initiated, it probably can be halted after the highest risk period passes.

Treatment is predicated on the assumption that recurrent seizures can be prevented with adequate medication. In the Hauser study,[2] treatment with antiepileptic medication was initially recommended for 80% of all cases. There did not appear to be a difference in recurrence rates between treated and untreated patients. This lack of effect may be explained by the study design, which was an observational and not an interventional analysis. Thus, compliance, uniformity of treatment, and other variables were not controlled. Only a few studies have examined treatment after a single seizure. One study randomized half of 397 patients aged 2 to 70 years to treatment with an antiepileptic drug after a single unprovoked generalized tonic-clonic seizure. The treated group had a calculated risk of seizure recurrence of 25% at 24 months, compared to 51% for the untreated persons.[12] Thus, limited clinical studies and intuition would suggest that treatment may prevent some but not all persons from having additional seizures.

In considering the issue of when to treat, social as well as therapeutic factors must be taken into account. For an adult, the most important question is that of driving a motor vehicle. In most cases, a single seizure has not been considered grounds for restricting driving, but the presence of epilepsy as demonstrated by the occurrence of two or more seizures subjects the patient to numerous restrictions. Thus, some patients, after reviewing the odds with their physician, elect to begin treatment after a single seizure. These decisions are difficult and should never be made unilaterally by the physician for the patient. Rather, the patient should be aware of the risks and benefits of the alternative strategies, and the key elements of the decision must be recorded in the medical record. In children, there may be less pressure to treat and the side effect profile may be less beneficial than in adults.[10,11] Also, identification of a specific epilepsy syndrome in a child can be useful in deciding whether to treat.

As shown in Figure 1, the steepest part of the recurrence rate curve is in the first 24 months, when the possibility of a second seizure is highest. Some physicians prefer to treat for 2 years in the case when the patient has no major risk factors but wishes to have protection from recurrence.

When to Stop Treatment

The decision to stop treatment must be made with the same consideration of the probability of recurrent seizures as in the decision to start treatment. Many older textbooks advised that treatment could be stopped after 2 years of seizure control. But this recommendation is not valid in the context of present knowledge of epileptic syndromes. As discussed briefly in Chapter 3, some epileptic syndromes are age-specific, and some patients mature to the stage of low risk. For example, children with benign epilepsy with centrotemporal spikes "outgrow" their seizures regardless of treatment. For other syndromes, however, there is a lifelong tendency for seizures to occur, and control of such seizures is not an indication that the disorder is in remission. A person with an arteriovenous malformation may achieve complete control for many years but remain at risk for seizures if medication is discontinued.

In one recent study, patients (mostly adults) who had been seizure-free for at least 4 years were asked to participate in a study of withdrawal of medication. Of 62 who elected to enter the withdrawal phase, 15 (24%) had a recurrent seizure. Of the 157 who declined to withdraw from medication, 10 (6%)

had a seizure.[13] In another study evaluating 1,013 patients who were seizure-free for at least 2 years, patients were prospectively randomized to withdrawal or continuation of treatment. In the continuing treatment group, 12% had subsequent seizures, while in the slow withdrawal group 41% had subsequent seizures.[14] The factors that appeared to be related to successful withdrawal were: single type of seizure; normal neurologic examination; normal IQ; and normal EEG following treatment. Thus, benefits of withdrawal (freedom from daily medication, reduction of side effects, decreased risk of teratogenic effects [Chapter 9]) must be balanced against a 20% to 30% probability of seizure recurrence (loss of job, possible injury). Whatever the decision, it must be made with the patient's full understanding of the risks involved. Medication should never be stopped abruptly because this may lead to withdrawal seizures or to status epilepticus. Rather, medications should be tapered over months, depending on the nature of the medication. Phenobarbital, with a long half-life and great potential for causing withdrawal seizures, should be withdrawn over many months, usually in increments of 25% of the initial dose. Phenytoin, carbamazepine, and valproate may be withdrawn over 6 to 10 weeks.

References

1. Hauser WA, Rich SS, Lee JR, et al: Risk of recurrent seizures after two unprovoked seizures. *N Engl J Med* 1998;338:429-434.

2. Hauser WA, Rich SS, et al: Seizure recurrence after a first unprovoked seizure: an extended follow-up. *Neurology* 1990;40:1163-1170.

3. Ewles RDC, Reynolds EH: Should people be treated after a first seizure? *Arch Neurol* 1988;45:490-491.

4. Annegers JF, Grabow JD, Groover RV, et al: Seizures after head trauma: a population study. *Neurology* 1980;30:683-689.

5. Annegers JF, Shirts SB, Hauser WA, et al: Risk of recurrence after an initial unprovoked seizure. *Epilepsia* 1986;27:43-50.

6. Hart RG, Easton JD: Seizure recurrence after a first, unprovoked seizure. *Arch Neurol* 1988;43:1289-1290.

7. Hauser WA, Ramiraz-Lassepas M, Rosenstein R: Risk for seizures and epilepsy following cerebrovascular insults. *Epilepsia* 1984;25:666. Abstract.

8. Hopkins A, Garman A, Clarke C: The first seizure in adult life. *Lancet* 1988;1:721-726.

9. Benedetti MD, Shinnar S, Cohen H, et al: Risk factors for epilepsy in children with cerebral palsy and/or mental retardation. *Epilepsia* 1986;27:614. Abstract.

10. Camfield PR, Camfield CS, Dooley JM, et al: Epilepsy after a first unprovoked seizure in childhood. *Neurology* 1985;35:1657-1660.

11. Shinnar S, Berg D, Moshe SL, et al: The risk of seizure recurrence following a first unprovoked seizure in childhood: a prospective study. *Pediatrics* 1990;85:1076-1085.

12. First Seizure Trial Group. Randomized clinical trial on the efficacy of antiepileptic drugs in reducing the risk of relapse after a first unprovoked tonic-clonic seizure. *Neurology* 1993;43:478-483.

13. Dean JC, Penry PK: Remission and relapse in chronic epilepsy. *Epilepsia* 1990;31(5):648. Abstract.

14. Chadwick D: Randomized study of AED withdrawal in patients in remission. Medical Research Council, AED Withdrawal Study Group. *Lancet* 1991;337:1175-1180.

Chapter 6

Principles of Treatment and Selection of an Antiepileptic Drug

The goal of treatment with antiepileptic drugs (AEDs) is to prevent the recurrence of seizures while avoiding side effects from the drugs. Treatment of epilepsy requires that both the physician and the patient understand the goals and time frame of treatment. Because no one can predict precisely when another seizure will occur, AEDs must be used so that therapeutic concentrations of the drug, its active metabolites, or its biochemical effector are present in the central nervous system for the period of risk. Moreover, because patients can have long intervals between seizures with no intervening symptoms, the issue of compliance becomes critical. The most common cause of treatment failure is noncompliance.[1]

As the basic mechanisms of the epilepsies and the actions of the AEDs become better known, a more rational approach to choosing drugs is emerging (Table 1). Phenytoin and carbamazepine have similar mechanisms of action; both inhibit rapid firing of use-dependent sodium channels. This effect would not cause significant alteration of the normal discharges of a neuron, but would diminish the capacity of abnormally discharging neurons to fire at excessive rates. Gabapentin, tiagabine, and vigabatrin have their major effect by enhancing gamma-aminobutyric acid (GABA) activity. Because GABA is the major inhibitory neurotransmitter in the CNS, these drugs may exert their action by reducing excitability. In general, both the sodium channel and GABA drugs are effective in localization-related epilepsy syndromes, and less effective or ineffective in generalized epilepsy syndromes. Other AEDs have multiple mechanisms, or less well defined mechanisms of action. Most of these AEDs are effective for the generalized epilepsies and for localization-related epilepsies. These AEDs include valproate, lamotrigine, tiagabine, phenobarbital, and zonisamide. Ethosuximide has been shown to have a single major mechanism of action, that of affecting calcium channels, and it is most effective for absence seizures

Table 1: Selecting AEDs Based on Classification of Epileptic Syndromes and Mechanisms of Action

Major Mechanism of Action	Drug	Effective for
Sodium channel drugs	carbamazepine* oxcarbazepine* phenytoin*	localization-related epilepsy
GABA enhance-ment drugs	gabapentin * tiagabine*	localization-related epilepsy
Mixed mechanisms (excitatory amino acid, sodium channel, GABA)	valproate lamotrigine	localization-related juvenile myoclonic
	felbamate valproate topiramate clonazepam lamotrigine	Lennox-Gastaut
	valproate clonazepam zonisamide	myoclonic
	valproate	absence
Calcium channel drugs	ethosuximide	absence
Unknown mechanism	levetiracetam	localization-related epilepsy

*may worsen Lennox-Gastaut, myoclonic

with little or no effect on partial or generalized tonic-clonic seizures. The mechanism of action of levetiracetam is unknown.

In adults, the most common seizure type is a partial seizure with secondary generalized, that is, localization-related epilepsy. One study comparing phenytoin and carbamazepine as initial therapy evaluated 70 patients (35 carbamazepine, 35 phenytoin) who were followed for 6 months to 2 years.[2] Of the patients without major side effects in whom efficacy of a single medication could be evaluated, control was obtained in 81.5% of the carbamazepine-treated group and in 85.8% of the phenytoin-treated group.

The largest prospective study to date (622 patients) of treatment efficacy was a multicenter Veterans Administration hospital (VAH) study that compared carbamazepine, phenytoin, primidone, and phenobarbital.[3] Patients were randomized to one of these four drugs, but were switched to another if toxicity occurred or if seizures were not controlled. Overall, the total seizure control was only 39% at 12 months and was similar with all the drugs tested (carbamazepine 47%, phenytoin 38%, phenobarbital 36%, and primidone 35%). The prognosis for complete control of tonic-clonic seizures with the four drugs was also similar (carbamazepine 48%, phenytoin 43%, phenobarbital 43%, and primidone 45%). Partial seizures were controlled with phenobarbital in 16%, with primidone in 15%, with phenytoin in 26%, and with carbamazepine in 43%. The difference in control between carbamazepine and phenytoin was not statistically significant but carbamazepine was statistically superior to phenobarbital and primidone.[3] Overall, for seizure control and toxicity, phenytoin and carbamazepine were similar, and both were superior to phenobarbital and primidone (Figure 1). These results have led to a decrease in use of the barbiturates.

One review of 20 trials evaluated 1,336 adult patients with newly diagnosed, presumed localization-related epilepsy. All the trials met the criterion of incorporating a prospective, randomized, double-blind design. But no significant difference was found in efficacy among the medications tested.[4] Thus, no well-controlled study has shown a significant difference in efficacy between carbamazepine and phenytoin, and choices must be made on factors other than efficacy alone.

Valproate has also been evaluated as treatment for complex-partial seizures. A recent VAH cooperative study found it to be slightly less effective than carbamazepine.[5] Another study, however, found no difference between phenytoin, valproate, and carbamazepine.[6]

Treatment should be started with a single drug. Some years ago, it was popular to initiate treatment with both phe-

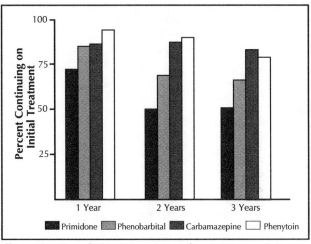

Figure 1—Cumulative percentage of patients remaining on initial drug (successfully treated) with primidone, phenobarbital, carbamazepine, and phenytoin, during 36 months of follow-up. (Adapted from information appearing in The New England Journal of Medicine.)[3]

nobarbital and phenytoin, based on the belief that these drugs had a synergistic action. However, the effect of these drugs in the central nervous system was shown to be additive and there is no longer a reason for initiating treatment with more than one medication.[7] Studies have shown that up to 80% of patients with new onset epilepsy can be successfully controlled with one medication.[8] However, if the first drug is not effective, another drug useful for the same category of seizures should be started. Some patients with intractable epilepsy will need more than one drug to control seizures.

Initiation of treatment can be done either by starting a maintenance dose or by using a loading dose followed by a maintenance dose (Figure 2). Most often, the treatment is started by using the maintenance dose. However, because five half-lives are needed to reach a steady-state level, loading is preferred in some instances. Knowledge of pharmacokinetic

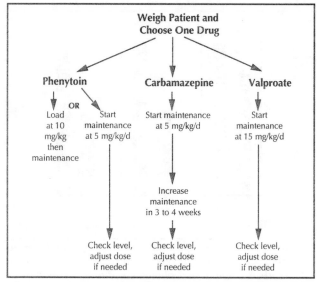

Figure 2—Initiation of treatment with the most widely used antiepileptic medications in adults. Doses as mg/kg/d may be larger for children or smaller for the elderly.

principles can be useful in developing initiation and maintenance strategies.

Initiation With Phenytoin

Because of its pK_a, phenytoin is not absorbed in the stomach, but must pass into the small intestine where the pH becomes alkaline. Thus, phenytoin absorption begins a few hours after administration and reaches its peak 6 to 12 hours later. Despite its slow absorption, the bioavailability of phenytoin is good; about 90% of an oral dose is absorbed.

Maintenance treatment with phenytoin in the adult can be started with 5 mg/kg/day. For many adults, this will be approximately 300 mg. Dosage adjustments should be made to meet individual requirements. If phenytoin is started as maintenance, it will take 5 to 7 days to reach steady-state concentration (five half-lives). But this may not be acceptable, especially if the patient is expected to be discharged from the hospital shortly, or if the patient has an acute series of seizures. In these cases, loading doses may be used.

Intravenous phenytoin has a volume of distribution (V_d) of 0.78 L/kg. Thus, an IV dose of 0.78 mg/kg will increase the blood level by 1.0 mg/L. Clinicians can tailor the dose to attain any specific desired blood level. For example, if one wishes to increase the blood level by 10 mg/L, one needs to give a dose of 7.8 mg/kg. For a 60-kg patient, this is approximately 480 mg. Fosphenytoin (Cerebyx®), a prodrug of phenytoin, has replaced parenteral Dilantin® and can be given either IV or IM for loading. For example, suppose a patient who has been well controlled by phenytoin concentrations of 15 mg/L has a breakthrough seizure. The patient is taken to the emergency department, where a concentration of 5 mg/L is recorded. Then the physician can give a dose of 7.8 mg/kg to restore the level to 15 mg/L. Studies have shown that oral doses of phenytoin of 1 mg/kg will raise the blood levels by 1 mg/kg. Partial loading may be useful if an increase in levels is needed.

During steady state, the dose must be sufficient to maintain the desired blood concentration. For an average adult, doses of 4 to 6 mg/kg per day are sufficient to maintain blood levels in the therapeutic range. For this reason, the patient's weight must be known. A standard dose of 300 mg/day may be sufficient for patients in the 60-kg range, but will be too high for patients weighing only 40 kg. On the other hand, patients weighing more than 100 kg (220 lb) will be underdosed if given 300 mg/day and instead need 500 mg/day.

Children are more rapid metabolizers of phenytoin than are adults. Children may need doses two or three times greater than adults on a mg-per-kg basis (8 to 10 mg/kg). Thus, a child weighing 30 kg may need 300 mg/day of phenytoin. The 30-mg capsules are useful for adjusting doses precisely (Table 2).

As patients grow older, there is a reduction in the cytochrome P-450 system, and doses used for adults may be too high for the elderly. Consequently, doses of 3 to 4 mg/kg/day may be more appropriate for the elderly. However, we lack good studies regarding dosing in this age group. Another issue is protein binding. Phenytoin is approximately 90% pro-

Table 2: Titration of Phenytoin

To attain the appropriate concentrations, use 100-mg and 30-mg doses of phenytoin to titrate in small increments. Dose increments of 10 mg are possible. Because there is a difference in mg of phenytoin between the capsule (sodium salt) and Infatabs®, titration with capsules rather than the 50-mg Infatabs is recommended. Some examples of combinations are:

Total daily dose	Number of 100 mg	Number of 30 mg
200	2	0
230	2	1
260	2	2
290	2	3
300	3	0
310	1	7
320	2	4
330	3	1
360	3	2
400	4	0

tein bound, and the usual methods for measuring this drug yield total concentrations, that is, both bound and unbound (free). The elderly may have lower albumin levels, so the total concentrations for them may be lower than for comparable "free" levels. For example, a patient with normal binding with a concentration of 15 mg/L would have a "free" level of 1.5 mg/L, and a bound level of 13.5 mg/L. However, if the binding is affected by low albumin, the unbound fraction may be 20% of the total, or 3.0 mg/L. This would be the equivalent of a total level of 30 mg/L in a patient with normal binding. Thus, if an elderly person exhibits symptoms of toxicity, but his or her total levels of phenytoin are in the therapeutic range, an unbound concentration should be obtained, or, more simply, the dose should be reduced to attain a lower steady-state level. In the elderly, total phenytoin concentrations of 5 to 10 mg/L may be sufficient.

Initiation With Carbamazepine

Carbamazepine dosage must be adjusted for each patient. Because it has a long half-life on initiation of therapy, doses of 200 mg b.i.d. are recommended for adults. Doses may be increased at weekly intervals by adding up to 200 mg/day using a t.i.d. or q.i.d. regimen until the best response is obtained. Doses should not generally exceed 1g/day in children 12 to 15 years of age, and should not exceed 1.2 g/day in patients 16 years of age or older. However, doses up to 2 g/day have been used in adults in some cases. Children 6 to 11 years of age should have an initial dose of 100 mg b.i.d., and doses can be increased at weekly intervals using a t.i.d. or q.i.d. regimen until the best response is obtained. Generally, doses of 5 to 8 mg/kg/day are sufficient during the first week of treatment but may need to be increased to 10 to 15 mg/kg/day with chronic use.

The half-life becomes shorter with chronic use because of autoinduction of carbamazepine metabolism, so the dosing interval may need to be increased to t.i.d. or q.i.d. Protein binding of carbamazepine is usually not clinically important. The major metabolite of carbamazepine, the 10,11-epoxide, also has antiepileptic properties and toxicity.

Carbamazepine use in the elderly has not been well studied. In general, doses may need to be lower on a mg/kg/day basis. Also, carbamazepine may interact with some medications used in the elderly.

Initiation With Valproate

The recommended initial dose of valproate is 15 mg/kg/day. Since valproate does not induce its own metabolism, doses do not need to be increased unless the patient is not obtaining full control. Doses may be increased at 1-week intervals by 5 to 10 mg/kg/day until seizures are controlled or until side effects preclude further increases. The maximum recommended dose is 60 mg/kg/day.

Monitoring Treatment

After AED therapy is initiated, treatment should be monitored for two important reasons: to evaluate the effectiveness of the AED, and to determine the drug's safety. Evaluating the effectiveness of treatment is best done by recording the patient's seizures accurately. It is recommended that patients with epilepsy record their seizures on a calendar so that an accurate assessment of effectiveness can be made. When a patient is doing well, with no seizures and no side effects, a blood level should be obtained to have a benchmark, or target, for that individual. This can be used in the future to determine control. If a patient has a breakthrough seizure and the level is significantly lower than the benchmark, noncompliance can be suspected. Then the physician can institute education and other means to foster compliance. If the level is at the benchmark, the target level can then be raised, on the conclusion that the seizure threshold is higher.

AEDs have been associated with rare, fatal aplastic anemia and hepatic failure. For this reason, it is necessary to obtain baseline values of hepatic and hematopoietic parameters. Some clinicians monitor these parameters every 3 to 6 months. Studies, however, indicate that the most cost-effective monitoring is done when patients are experiencing symptoms (Chapter 9).

It is useful to measure AED levels at least annually to assure that compliance is being maintained and to confirm that there have been no significant changes in metabolism of the drugs. This is particularly important if the physician is taking responsibility for certifying eligibility for the patient's driving privileges.

References

1. Leppik IE, Schmidt D: Summary of the First International Workshop on Compliance in Epilepsy. *Epilepsy Res* 1988;1(suppl):179-182.

2. Ramsay RE, Wilder BJ, Berger JR, et al: A double-blind study comparing carbamazepine with phenytoin as initial seizure therapy in adults. *Neurology* 1975;33:904-910.

3. Mattson RH, Cramer JA, Collins JF, et al: Comparison of carbamazepine, phenobarbital, phenytoin, and primidone in partial and secondarily generalized tonic-clonic seizures. *N Engl J Med* 1985;313:145-151.

4. Treiman DM: Efficacy and safety of antiepileptic drugs: a review of controlled trials. *Epilepsia* 1987;28(suppl 3):S1-S8.

5. Mattson RH, et al: Valproate vs carbamazepine for seizures, a comparison of valproate with carbamazepine for the treatment of complex partial seizures and secondarily generalized tonic-clonic seizures in adults. *N Engl J Med* 1992;327(11):765.

6. Callaghan N, Kenny RA, O'Neill B, et al: A prospective study between carbamazepine, phenytoin, and sodium valproate as mono-

therapy in previously untreated and recently diagnosed patients with epilepsy. *J Neurol Neurosurg Psychiatry* 1985;48:639-644.

7.   Leppik IE, Sherwin AL: Anticonvulsant activity of phenobarbital and phenytoin in combination. *J Pharmacol Exp Ther* 1977;200:570-576.

8.   Reynolds EH, Chadwick D, Galbraith AW: One drug (phenytoin) in the treatment of epilepsy. *Lancet* 1976;1:923-926.

Chapter 7

Antiepileptic Drugs (AEDs)

T his chapter examines in detail information about the specific attributes of the antiepileptic drugs (AEDs). It summarizes each drug's actions and uses, pharmacokinetics, doses and preparations, adverse reactions, and common drug

Table 1:	Doses and Plasma Concentrations of Standard Antiepileptic Drugs	
	Average Daily Maintenance Dose	
Drug	**Adults (mg)**	**Adults (mg/kg)**
Carbamazepine	600 mg-1.2 g	5-15
Clonazepam	2-6 mg	0.1-0.2
Ethosuximide	500 mg-2.0 g	15-40
Felbamate	1800-3600	
Gabapentin	900-3600	
Lamotrigine	150-1200	
Levetiracetam	1000-3000	20-40 mg/kg
Oxcarbazepine	600-2400	
Phenobarbital	120-250 mg	2-3
Phenytoin	300-400 mg	4-6
Primidone	750 mg-1.5 g	8-16
Tiagabine	20-100	
Topiramate	200-600	
Valproate	750 mg-1.0 g (monotherapy)	15-25 (monotherapy)
	1.5-3.0 g (combination therapy)	30-60 (combination therapy)
Zonisamide	200-600	

*Concentrations are reported as µg/mL by some laboratories, but mg/L is the preferred unit and will be used in this book.
1 µg/mL= 1 mg/L

interactions. Table 1 is a summary of the doses and levels of the AEDs.

History of Antiepileptic Medications

The first effective drug for treatment of epileptic seizures was bromide. In 1857, Locock, in a discussion of a paper on the etiology of seizures, disclosed that he had had remarkable success using bromide in female patients with intractable epilepsy. His experience was confirmed by others, and soon tons of bromide were being used as primary therapy for epilepsy.

Children (mg/kg)	Usually Effective Plasma Concentrations (mg/L)*
15-30	4-12
0.1-0.2	0.02-0.08
15-40	40-100
15-45	30-100
15-45	4-20
	4-20
	5-40
	4-12▲
3-5	15-40
6-8	10-20
10-25	5-12
	100-300**
	20-50
15-20 (monotherapy)	40-120
30-100 (combination therapy)	
	20-40

**ng/mL
▲MHD (10-monohydroxy metabolite)

Table 2: Antiepileptic Drugs Marketed in the United States

Year Introduced	Name	Year Introduced	Name
1912	phenobarbital	1975	clonazepam
1935	mephobarbital	1978	valproate
1938	phenytoin	1981	clorazepate
1947	mephenytoin	1993	felbamate
1949	paramethadione		gabapentin
1951	phenacemide	1994	lamotrigine
1953	phensuximide	1996	fosphenytoin
1954	primidone	1996	topiramate
1957	methsuximide	1997	tiagabine
1957	ethotoin	1999	levetiracetam
1960	ethosuximide	2000	oxcarbazepine
1968	diazepam		zonisamide
1974	carbamazepine		

Before the introduction of bromide, almost every conceivable potion, diet, and ritual had been used without significant benefit. Although effective for controlling seizures, bromide's side effects are considerable and include sedation, depression, skin eruptions, and gastrointestinal distress. For more than 60 years, bromide was the only effective substance known for the treatment of epilepsy. Because it was a prominent side effect of bromide, sedation was considered by many to be essential for anticonvulsant effect. Based on this concept, Hauptmann proposed using phenobarbital for the treatment of epilepsy in 1912. For the next 25 years, epilepsy was treated with drugs associated with slowing of mentation, and in retrospect, much of the belief that persons with epilepsy were mentally subnormal may have been a result of the treatment rather than the disorder. Today, it is difficult to imagine that substances to treat illnesses could be given to humans before being thoroughly tested in animals for safety and efficacy, but this had been the case for millennia. It was only in the early part of this century that the scientific community and the public began to see the value of animal testing prior to exposure in humans.[1]

The work of Merritt and Putnam with phenytoin demonstrated that the use of an animal model of seizures was an efficient way to screen a large number of compounds for antiepileptic effectiveness. Their work also showed that sedation and depression were not essential for anticonvulsant effect.[2] The subsequent introduction of antiepileptic drugs was rapid. From 1946 to 1978, 17 other substances were approved for marketing in the United States (Table 2). Some have been withdrawn because of toxicity and many of the others have been found to have only limited utility and are infrequently used.

From 1961 through 1973, no major new drugs for epilepsy were marketed in the United States, although carbamazepine, valproate, and other agents were being used in other countries. Carbamazepine was approved for marketing in the United States in 1974. Valproate was approved in 1978, and then there were no new major drugs approved for the treatment of epilepsy until 1993. Nevertheless, there were significant advances in the use of antiepileptic drugs. This knowledge was acquired by the emergence of new technology to measure antiepileptic drug concentrations in the blood. Previous dosage schedules that were derived solely from clinical experience were replaced by dosage schedules based on pharmacokinetic principles. Additionally, it became possible to determine patient compliance with prescribed therapy.

Another important development was the acceptance of an international classification of epileptic seizures and the epilepsy syndromes (Table 1, Chapter 2, and Table 1, Chapter 3). This made the evaluation of current and new drugs more rational. Also, developments in the knowledge of the mechanism of action and of the biochemical mechanisms underlying the genesis of seizures have opened up new avenues of drug development.

Starting in the late 1970s, a renewed interest occurred in developing new drugs for epilepsy treatment in the United States. The Epilepsy Branch of the National Institutes of Health began a comprehensive system for screening promising compounds in animal models of epilepsy. More than 27,000 compounds have been screened, and from these a few were promising enough to warrant testing in humans. During the past decade, more than 18 compounds have been tested in humans in the United States. Under present FDA regulations that require both efficacy and safety to be demonstrated in scientifically valid clinical trials in hundreds of patients, much effort has been expended to develop new drugs or new formulations of presently marketed compounds. The FDA approved felbamate and gabapentin in 1993, lamotrigine in 1994, topiramate in 1996, tiagabine in 1997, levetiracetam in 1999, and oxcarbazepine and zonisamide in 2000.

Other new drugs are in clinical trials in the United States.

Although extensive phase 2 and phase 3 testing is performed on all new drugs before FDA approval, this clinical testing of a few thousand patients is not sufficient to exclude rare and idiosyncratic side effects. In the case of felbamate, extensive animal and clinical testing in more than 2,000 subjects did not reveal any risk for bone marrow suppression. Only after a year of use and prescriptions to more than 100,000 patients did the strong association emerge (approximately 1 in 5,000 patients per year). We cannot now predict what other problems may arise over time with these newer compounds. However, gabapentin and lamotrigine have been used in well over 400,000 patients worldwide and we can only hope that the felbamate experience will not be repeated.

Baseline, CBC, reticulocyte counts, and liver function tests should be done at initiation of treatment with any antiepileptic drug new to the patient. Although many of the new drugs are water soluble, parenteral preparations have not yet been approved.

Pharmacokinetic properties influence how drugs should be dosed; in general, the dose interval should be shorter than the half-life. There is a considerable change in half-life with age: children have the shortest, adults longer, and elderly and newborns the longest (Table 3).

Drug interactions are a major problem. Investigators have recently increased our knowledge of the cytochrome P-450 system, and have characterized many of its isoenzymes and their substrates.[3] By knowing which isoenzymes each drug uses, it is now possible to predict possible interactions. The CYP 3A4 isoenzyme accounts for 60% to 70% of enzymes in the liver and gut. It has numerous substrates, including many AEDs, as well as oral contraceptives and other hormones. It is induced by carbamazepine, ethosuximide, oxcarbazepine, phenobarbital, phenytoin, and primidone.

These substrate concentrations can be lowered by these AEDs or, if present in high concentrations, these substrates, can inhibit AEDs. Table 4 gives a list of some of the important interactions. The FDA is now requiring isoenzyme profiling of all new drugs, so clinicians should review the latest package inserts. Because the field of isoenzyme profiling is so new, information about profiles is still somewhat preliminary and subject to change as more information becomes available. Drug interactions are a particularly important problem in the elderly, many of whom require other medications (Table 4). Drug interactions from AEDs, although somewhat predictable, will vary from patient to patient. Generally, a drug that stimulates hepatic metabolism will lower concentrations of other drugs that use the liver for detoxification. However, by blocking some enzyme systems, drugs can also increase the concentrations by inhibiting metabolism.

A general statement regarding AEDs can be made. Phenobarbital is a very potent inducer of many isoenzymes, and interactions are very common. Phenytoin is almost as strong, and carbamazepine, and to a lesser degree oxcarbazepine, have broad inducing effects. Almost all AED concentrations are decreased by these four. Most of the newer drugs have much lower or no effect on inducing or inhibiting isoenzymes of the P-450 system. Gabapentin and levetiracetam are primarily renally excreted and thus have no effect on, and are not affected by, other drugs. For highly protein-bound drugs, displacement from binding sites will lower the total serum concentration without necessarily affecting the biological activity. This is a special concern for phenytoin and valproate, which are greater than 90% protein bound. In addition to their metabolic interaction, displacement from protein-binding sites will yield lower total concentration measurements, which can be misleading.

Carbamazepine: Action and Uses

Carbamazepine (Tegretol®) is effective alone or with other AEDs in partial seizures, especially complex partial seizures, in generalized tonic-clonic seizures, and in combinations of these seizure types. It is ineffective for absence, myoclonic, and atonic seizures. Carbamazepine may exacerbate some generalized seizures with spike-and-wave EEG patterns in children.[4]

Comparative clinical trial data indicate that carbamazepine is better tolerated than phenobarbital and primidone in simple and complex partial seizures, but individual responses vary.[5]

Table 3: Pharmacokinetic Data on Antiepileptic Drugs

Drug	Time to Steady State (Days)	Plasma Half-Life (Hours)	
		Adults	
		Mean	Range
Carbamazepine	21–28	10–20[a]	5–26
Clonazepam	6		18–50
Ethosuximide	7–10	52–56	40–60
Felbamate	5-10	15-24	
Gabapentin	1	4-6	4-10[d]
Lamotrigine	4-15	15-60	30-40 (monotherapy) 50-70 (with valproate) 15-30 (with inducers)
Levetiracetam	1	8-10	
Oxcarbazepine	3	8-10	
Phenobarbital	>21	96	53–140
Phenytoin	6–8[b]	20–30[c]	8–59
Primidone	4–7	15	4–22
Topiramate	5-10	20-24	
Tiagabine	1	4-7	
Valproate	1–4		12–16 (mono-therapy)
		8	5–10 (poly-therapy)
Zonisamide	5-15	24-60	

[a]Initially the average half-life is 30 to 35 hours; values listed are after autoinduction.
[b]May be 2 to 3 weeks if plasma concentrations are above 20 mg/L.
[c]Half-life increases with dose.

Children		Volume Distribution (L/kg)	Plasma Protein Binding (%)	Elimination Site
Mean	Range			
8–14	3–25	0.8–1.4	75	hepatic
	22–33	1.5–4.4	85	hepatic
30–36	15–68	0.67	<5	hepatic
			low	hepatic and renal
			none	renal
			low	hepatic
			very low	hepatic and renal
			low	hepatic
67–72	37–133	0.5–1.0	40–60	hepatic and renal
		0.5–1.0	90	hepatic
10		0.8	20	hepatic and renal
			low	hepatic and renal
			low	hepatic
	8–12 (mono-therapy)	0.15	80–94[e]	hepatic
8	5–9 (poly-therapy)			
			low	hepatic and renal

[d]Pharmacodynamic half-life may be longer.
[e]Percent bound decreases as total plasma concentration increases above 75-100 mg/L.

This drug is increasingly preferred to phenobarbital in pediatric patients because it appears to have less effect than phenobarbital on cognition and behavior.

Pharmacokinetics

Oral absorption of carbamazepine is variable; peak plasma concentrations occur in 4 to 12 hours after use of solid dosage forms. Bioavailability is estimated at 85%, but may be less when the drug is taken with meals. Rate of absorption may vary with different prescriptions. There are now two sustained-release preparations, Tegretol®-XR and Carbatrol®. With monotherapy, the usual effective plasma concentration is 4 to 12 mg/L, but higher concentrations may be required in some patients to control seizures. With concomitant use of other AEDs, low concentrations may be associated with toxicity.

Carbamazepine is metabolized in the liver to its 10,11-epoxide. This compound has both anticonvulsant and toxic effects.[6] Carbamazepine induces its own metabolism; as a result, the usual initial half-life (18 to 35 hours) is reduced considerably after 3 or 4 weeks of administration. Children metabolize carbamazepine faster than adults do and they need larger doses (Table 1). Because of autoinduction of metabolism, plasma concentrations should be monitored during the first month of treatment. Also, because concomitant use of phenytoin or phenobarbital may further induce this metabolic pathway, significantly larger doses of carbamazepine often are required when it is used in combination. Because of its short half-life and rapid absorption, wide variations may occur between peak and trough levels. To overcome this, extended-release forms, Tegretol®-XR and Carbatrol®, were developed.

Dosage and Administration

Oral: Children 6 to 12 years, 100 mg twice daily on the first day. The amount can be increased by 100 mg daily at appropriate intervals (usually 1 to 2 weeks) and given in three or four divided doses until the desired response is obtained (usual maximum dose, 1 g). The usual daily maintenance dose is 400 to 800 mg (15 to 30 mg/kg); the frequency of administration must be individualized. For children 4 to 6 years, 10 to 20 mg/kg in two or three divided doses is warranted, increased by up to 100 mg daily at weekly intervals, as needed and tolerated. The usual maintenance dose is 250 to 350 mg a day (usual maximum dose, 400 mg). For children under 4 years, an initial dose of 20 to 60 mg is recommended.[7]

For adults and adolescents, initially 400 mg should be divided into two doses on the first day, increased by 200 mg daily at appropriate intervals (usually 1 to 2 weeks) and administered in three or four divided doses. The usual daily maintenance dose is 600 mg to 1.2 g in monotherapy, but may be as high as 2.0 g in combination therapy. Elderly patients metabolize carbamazepine more slowly and therefore will need lower doses.

Carbamazepine suspension may be given through a nasogastric tube, but this requires careful flushing.

Intravenous and intramuscular: not available.

Rectal suspension: can be used for rectal administration.

Generic: tablets 200 mg; chewable tablets 100 mg.

Tegretol® (Novartis): tablets 200 mg; chewable tablets 100 mg; suspension 100 mg/5 mL.

Tegretol® XR: tablets 100, 200, 400 mg.

Carbatrol® (Shire): 200, 300 mg extended-release capsules

Adverse Reactions and Precautions

Baseline blood and platelet counts, urinalysis, and hepatic and renal function studies should be performed before initiating treatment with carbamazepine. But excessively frequent and specialized monitoring is unwarranted and costly (see Chapter 9). Careful attention to new symptoms is probably equally effective in preventing serious complications.[8] Dermatologic reactions such as pruritic and erythematous rashes and urticaria have been reported in 2% to 4% of patients. Less common but more serious are Stevens-Johnson syndrome, photosensitivity, exfoliative dermatitis, erythema multiforme, erythema nodosum, and aggravation of systemic lupus erythematosus. Petechiae, pallor, weakness, fever, or infection may be symptoms of a potentially fatal reaction and patients should be instructed to contact their physician immediately.

Less serious side effects that occur during early treatment with carbamazepine are drowsiness, dizziness, lightheadedness, diplopia, ataxia, nausea, and vomiting. These usually subside spontaneously within a week or after a reduction in dose. Less common neurologic reactions include confusion, headache, fatigue, blurred vision, oculomotor disturbances, dysphasia, abnormal involuntary movements, peripheral neuritis and paresthesias, depression with agitation, talkativeness, nystagmus, and tinnitus.

Gastrointestinal reactions include gastric distress and abdominal pain, diarrhea, constipation, and anorexia. Dryness of the mouth, glossitis, and stomatitis also occur.

Transient leukopenia occurs in approximately 10% of patients treated with carbamazepine, but discontinuance of the drug usually is not required. Other hematopoietic reactions (eosinophilia, leukocytosis, purpura, and thrombocytopenia) are rare. Although very uncommon, these reactions may be fatal. Because their onset is gradual and reversible when the drug is discontinued, patients should be advised to notify their physician if fever, sore throat, aphthous stomatitis, easy bruising, petechial or purpuric hemorrhage, or other signs of hematologic toxicity appear.

Carbamazepine has an antidiuretic hormonelike effect that may be troublesome, particularly in cardiac or elderly patients. Mild, asymptomatic hyponatremia is a common laboratory finding.[9] Serious water intoxication with sodium concentrations below 120 mEq/L—and characterized by confusion, lethargy, neurologic dysfunction, and seizures—is uncommon.

Cardiovascular, genitourinary, metabolic, hepatic, and other reactions have been reported rarely. These include aggravation of hypertension or ischemic heart disease, arrhythmias, hypotension, syncope, edema, congestive heart failure, recurrence of thrombophlebitis, urinary frequency, acute urinary retention, albuminuria, glycosuria, elevated blood urea nitrogen levels, microscopic deposits in the urine, impotence, cholestatic and hepatocellular jaundice, fever and chills, myalgia and arthralgia, leg cramps, and conjunctivitis.

Drug Interactions

Approximately 75% of carbamazepine is bound to plasma albumin, but this is not clinically significant. As a result of enzyme induction, carbamazepine increases the hepatic metabolism of many drugs (Table 4). Valproate has a variable effect on carbamazepine steady-state concentrations and decreases carbamazepine epoxide metabolism, which may have therapeutic or toxic significance.[6] Carbamazepine concentrations are markedly increased by erythromycin and propoxyphene hydrochloride. Other drugs may have lesser effects. Carbamazepine also may reduce the plasma concentration and therapeutic response to corticosteroids or thyroid hormones. The combination of carbamazepine and lithium may increase the risk of neurotoxicity.

Phenytoin and Fosphenytoin: Actions and Uses

Phenytoin (Dilantin®) is useful in generalized tonic-clonic, complex partial, and simple partial seizures. Comparative data from clinical trials indicate that phenytoin is better tolerated than phenobarbital and primidone.[5] It is ineffective in absence, myoclonic, and atonic seizures and is not recommended for the treatment of epileptic syndromes in which absence seizures or myoclonus are present. Intravenous fosphenytoin is an effective treatment for status epilepticus and can be used as the initial drug to manage recurrent seizures.

Pharmacokinetics

Bioavailability of phenytoin averages 85% to 90% with most preparations. However, time to peak plasma concentration is variable and increases with the dose, but normally occurs within 4 to 8 hours for prompt-release capsules, and somewhat later for the extended-release preparations. Plasma protein binding is 90%. Phenytoin is eliminated almost entirely by hepatic metabolism. Oxidative metabolism proceeds via an epoxide intermediate, which probably represents the rate-limiting step.

Plasma concentrations are not related linearly to the daily dose because of saturable nonlinear metabolism, and small increases in dose may greatly increase the plasma concentration. Plasma concentrations of 10 to 20 mg/L are usually effective. However, higher or lower concentrations may sometimes be therapeutic and clinical outcome should determine the appropriate level for each patient.

Since phenytoin demonstrates nonlinear elimination kinetics, clearance and apparent half-life are dose-dependent. However, there is significant intersubject variability in phenytoin metabolism. Methods used to guide phenytoin dose adjustments include: graphic, which employs a linear transformation of the Michaelis-Menten equation; nomograms; estimates using population clearance values; and bayesian procedures. A simple method using a semilogarithmic plot of steady-state drug concentrations versus corresponding maintenance doses also has been described.[10]

Table 4: Clinically Significant Drug Interactions

Drug/Isoenzyme	Levels Increased by[a]

Carbamazepine
  CYP 3A4/5 sub+ind
  CYP 2D6 ind
  CYP 2C9 ind
  CYP 1A2 ind
  CYP 2C19 ind
	erythromycin
	clarithromycin
	isoniazid
	propoxyphene
	troleandomycin
	cimetidine
	danazol
	diltiazem
	verapamil
	fluoxetine
	sertraline
	fluvoxamine
	indinavir
	grapefruit juice

Note: The isoenzyme information is being developed rapidly and is subject to change.

| Phenytoin
  CYP 2C9, 2C19 sub+ind
  CYP 3A4/5 ind
  CYP 2D6 ind
  CYP 2A2 ind | **topiramate**
chloramphenicol
cimetidine
dicumarol
disulfiram
isoniazid
phenylbutazone
sulfonamides
trimethoprim
amiodarone
allopurinol
chlorpheniramine
fluoxetine
fluvoxamine
ranitidine
omeprazole
fluconazole |

AEDs are in bold
[a] inhibits metabolism of AEDs   sub = enzyme substrate
[b] induces metabolism of AEDs   blk = enzyme blocker (inhibitor)
ind = enzyme inducer

| | Effect on Other Drugs | |
Levels Decreased by[b]	Increases	Decreases
phenobarbital[1] phenytoin[1]		clonazepam ethosuximide primidone valproate topiramate phenytoin[1] phenobarbital[1] oral contraceptives disopyramide rifampin ketoconazole meperidine warfarin tacrolimus protease inhibitors trazodone quinidine
carbamazepine[1] phenobarbital[1] valproate[1] diazoxide antineoplastics loxepine rifampin		topiramate carbamazepine[1] phenobarbital[1] primidone[1] valproate[1] oral contraceptives disopyramide quinidine ketoconazole itraconazole etoposide corticosteroids warfarin trazodone cyclosporine tacrolimus protease inhibitors methadone propafenone theophylline

[1] Variable effects (increase, decrease, no change) reported

(continued on next page)

Table 4: Clinically Significant Drug Interactions *(continued)*

Drug/Isoenzyme	Levels Increased by[a]
Valproate 2C9 blk	
Ethosuximide CYP 3A4 sub	
Phenobarbital/Primidone CYP 1A2, 2B6, 2C8-10, 3A4, 3A5-7 ind	
Gabapentin no hepatic metabolism	
Lamotrigine	**valproate**
Felbamate CYP 2C19 blk	
Topiramate CYP 3A sub	
Tiagabine	
Levetiracetam no significant hepatic metabolism	
Oxcarbazepine CYP 3A4, 5-7 ind CYP 2C19 blk	
Zonisamide CYP 2C19 sub CYP 2D6 sub CYP 3A4 sub	

AEDs are in bold
[a] inhibits metabolism of AEDs
[b] induces metabolism of AEDs
[c] AEDs inhibit metabolism of

Effect on Other Drugs

Levels Decreased by[b]	Increases[c]	Decreases[d]
carbamazepine phenobarbital primidone phenytoin salicylates	lamotrigine phenobarbital carbamazepine[3] carbamazepine epoxide	phenytoin[2] ethosuximide[1]
carbamazepine phenobarbital phenytoin primidone		
phenytoin carbamazepine		(same list as phenytoin)
phenytoin carbamazepine		
phenytoin phenobarbital carbamazepine	phenytoin valproate carbamazepine epoxide	carbamazepine
phenytoin carbamazepine	phenytoin	
phenytoin carbamazepine phenobarbital		
phenytoin carbamazepine phenobarbital	phenytoin	oral contraceptives (probably same list as **carbamazepine**)
carbamazepine phenytoin phenobarbital		

[d] AEDs induce metabolism of
1 Variable effects (increase, decrease, no change) reported
2 Variable effects on free and total plasma concentrations
3 Increases the carbamazepine epoxide/carbamazepine ratio

Phenytoin's nonlinear kinetics accentuate the variations in blood levels caused by alterations in the rates of dissolution and absorption among the various dosage forms and products.[11] Thus, phenytoin plasma concentrations may differ significantly from one product to another and blood levels must be monitored when product substitutions are made. Thus, in calculating cost-savings in switching, the costs of laboratory testing and medical care costs must be considered.[11]

The plasma concentration of free phenytoin can be increased by hyperbilirubinemia (eg, in neonates, in those with liver disease), hypoalbuminemia (eg, in the elderly, in those with liver disease), and uremia. Febrile illnesses may markedly increase the clearance of phenytoin, leading to lowered plasma concentrations.[12] Phenytoin plasma concentrations also may be reduced by concurrent enteral feeding.[13]

Dosage and Administration

Oral: The dosage must be individualized according to the patient's response and to the drug concentrations. Phenytoin may be administered in divided doses (but does not need to be dosed more than twice daily). In adults, once-daily administration is usually sufficient to maintain plasma concentrations in the therapeutic range once steady state has been achieved. It also improves compliance. However, once-daily dosage may not be practical in patients who tend to miss doses.

For adults, initially 300 mg daily is recommended in two divided doses; the maintenance dose is usually 4 to 6 mg/kg/day. Incremental increases can be made using 30-mg capsules. Formulation differences between tablet and capsules may cause problems in precise dose titration. The tablets (free acid phenytoin) contain 8% more phenytoin than the phenytoin sodium capsules. Dosing regimens for the elderly have not been well established but are usually 3 to 4 mg/kg/day lower than those in adults.

For children, maintenance doses may need to be higher, 7 mg/kg/day or more.

Phenytoin suspension may be given through a nasogastric tube, but this must be flushed well and clamped after administration.

Intravenous: Phenytoin is very water insoluble, and a mixture of 40% propylene glycol (antifreeze), and 10% alcohol,

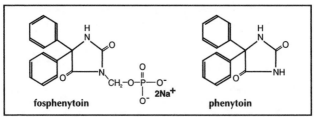

Figure 1—*Chemical formulae for fosphenytoin and for phenytoin.*

adjusted to a pH of 12 with sodium hydroxide (Drano®) is needed to make it soluble. It must be administered slowly to avoid hypotension or cardiac arrhythmias. Also, it is very sclerosing, and must be given through an intracatheter into a large vein. Leakage from the injection site into the subcutaneous tissue can cause necrosis. To circumvent these problems, fosphenytoin (Cerebyx®), a prodrug, has been developed. It consists of a phosphate group that is joined to the phenytoin molecule by an ester bond (Figure 1). This molecule is rapidly and completely converted in vivo to phenytoin with a half-life of 8 to 12 minutes. Thus, within 20 to 30 minutes, almost all of the fosphenytoin has been converted to phenytoin in the body. The advantages of this preparation are that it is formulated in aqueous solution near normal pH and without propylene glycol or alcohol. It is well tolerated and does not cause venous sclerosis. Also, it can be administered without the complications associated with the present preparation.[14] Dilantin® solution is no longer available; it has been replaced by Cerebyx®.

Intramuscular: The phenytoin preparation now in use should not be given intramuscularly because it precipitates, forming painful and insoluble crystals. However, fosphenytoin is readily absorbed after IM injection. It causes little discomfort.[14] The availability of this IM preparation has made it possible to replace oral phenytoin in situations where a patient is NPO without resorting to IV administration. Also, this preparation may be used when a patient has had some seizures and has a low phenytoin level. The situation may not be urgent enough to require IV loading, but the oral preparation does not reach peak absorption for 8 to 12 hours. The use of fosphenytoin IM would be useful in this situation.

Rectal: Phenytoin is not absorbed rectally.

Phenytoin (free acid):

Generic: Suspension 125 mg/ 5 mL (alcohol < 0.6%).

Dilantin® (Parke-Davis): Suspension 125 mg/5 mL (alcohol < 0.6%); tablets (chewable) 50 mg.

Phenytoin sodium:

Generic: Capsules 100 mg.

Dilantin® (Parke-Davis): Capsules (extended) 30 mg and 100 mg.

Phenytoin solution:

Generic: Solution 50 mg/mL in propylene glycol 40%, alcohol 10%, pH adjusted to 11-12.

(Dilantin® [Parke-Davis]: discontinued in 1997.)

Fosphenytoin solution:

Cerebyx® 75 mg/mL (equivalent to 50 mg/mL of phenytoin) in 2-mL and 5-mL vials.

Adverse Reactions and Precautions

Phenytoin produces little or no sedation at concentrations below 20 mg/L. Plasma concentrations above 20 mg/L may be associated with concentration-dependent symptoms of toxicity: nystagmus, ataxia, and lethargy. However, in the absence of symptoms, doses should not be decreased if levels are above 20 mg/L.

Skin eruptions occur in approximately 8% of patients but are rarely serious and are unrelated to the initial dosage or to the plasma concentration.[15] Peripheral neuropathy may develop after years of use. Mild gingival hyperplasia may be seen on careful oral examinations in 20% to 50% of patients. Scrupulous oral hygiene prevents secondary inflammation and severe hyperplasia is uncommon. Hypertrichosis and hirsutism are less common.

Rare but serious idiosyncratic reactions include hepatitis, bone-marrow depression, systemic lupus erythematosus, Stevens-Johnson syndrome, and lymphadenopathy. These often disappear after therapy is discontinued. A few cases of lymphoma and Hodgkin's disease have been reported.

Drug Interactions

Phenytoin may reduce the plasma concentration of carbamazepine, valproate, ethosuximide, and primidone by enzyme induction. Phenytoin and phenobarbital exert variable, reciprocal effects. Valproate displaces phenytoin from protein-binding sites but inhibits metabolism. Total plasma concentrations may be decreased, but the unbound (free) may change little or may increase. Other drugs that may displace phenytoin include phenylbutazone, salicylates, and tolbutamide. The total plasma concentration of phenytoin may decrease, but the actual free concentration may be relatively unchanged because of the increase in the free fraction.

Drugs that significantly increase the plasma concentration of phenytoin include chloramphenicol, cimetidine, dicumarol, disulfiram, isoniazid, sulfonamides, and trimethoprim. Amiodarone, allopurinol, chlorpheniramine, and trazodone may possibly increase the plasma phenytoin concentration. Folic acid, prolonged ingestion of alcohol, and rifampin may decrease the phenytoin plasma concentration. In patients with tuberculosis, the effects of rifampin and isoniazid may cancel each other when these drugs are used with phenytoin. Certain antineoplastic agents (bleomycin, cisplatin, vinblastine) may also reduce plasma concentrations of phenytoin.

Phenytoin is a relatively potent enzyme inducer and may decrease the effectiveness of oral anticoagulants, certain antibiotics (doxycycline, rifampin, and chloramphenicol), oral contraceptives, antiarrhythmic agents (disopyramide, mexiletine, quinidine) digitoxin, analgesics (meperidine, methadone), cyclosporine, corticosteroids, and theophylline. Pharmacologically, phenytoin has been reported to impair blood pressure control by dopamine and to decrease the response to nondepolarizing skeletal muscle relaxants.

Valproate: Actions and Uses

Valproate (valproic acid [Depakene®] and divalproex sodium [Depakote®]) control absence, myoclonic, and tonic seizures in generalized, idiopathic epilepsy. It is most useful in typical absence seizures. Valproate is as effective as ethosuximide in patients with absence seizures alone and is variably effective in atypical absence seizures. Valproate is the drug of choice for patients with both absence and generalized tonic-clonic seizures.

Retrospective comparisons of valproate with carbamazepine or phenytoin in the treatment of partial and secondarily generalized seizures indicate that valproate is equally effective. But a prospective, controlled multicenter trial of carbamazepine and valproate in partial seizures indicated carbamazepine to be slightly more effective.[16]

Valproate is the drug of choice in myoclonic epilepsy, with or without generalized tonic-clonic seizures that begin in adolescence or early adulthood. Valproate usually controls photosensitive myoclonus and is also effective in the treatment of benign myoclonic epilepsy, postanoxic myoclonus, and, with clonazepam, in severe progressive myoclonic epilepsy that is characterized by tonic-clonic seizures. It also may be preferred in certain stimulus-sensitive (reflex, startle) epilepsies.

Although valproate may be effective for infantile spasms, it is relatively contraindicated in children whose spasms are caused by hyperglycinemia or other underlying metabolic (mitochondrial) abnormalities.

In general, atonic and akinetic seizures in patients with Lennox-Gastaut syndrome are difficult to control, but valproate is an effective drug of choice for treatment of these mixed seizure types.

Pharmacokinetics

Valproic acid (Depakene®) is absorbed rapidly and completely in the stomach after oral administration; peak plasma concentrations usually occur within 0.5 to 2 hours. The delayed-release tablet preparation, divalproex sodium (Depakote®), reaches peak plasma concentrations 3 to 6 hours after ingestion. A slow-release form (Depakote® Sprinkle) is also available. Total availability of valproate is unaffected by food.

The plasma protein binding of valproate is saturable within the usual therapeutic range (approximately 90% at 75 mg/L). Usual effective plasma concentrations range from 50 to 100 mg/L, but higher concentrations exceeding 150 mg/L may be required and tolerated in some patients. With a daily dose of more than 50 mg/kg, total plasma concentrations may not increase proportionately because both clearance and free fraction increase. Daily fluctuations in free fraction and clearance also occur as a result of displacement by free fatty acids or circadian influences.

Valproate is eliminated almost exclusively by hepatic metabolism. Its metabolic fate is complex. A variety of conjugation and oxidative processes are involved, including pathways (eg, beta oxidation) normally reserved for endogenous fatty acids. As the dose is increased, mitochondrial beta oxidation occurs. In mitochondrial pathways, sequential use of acetyl-CoA and carnitine may interfere with intermediary metabolism. Rarely, valproate may induce secondary carnitine deficiency.

Metabolites may contribute to both antiepileptic and hepatotoxic effects. One metabolite, the 2-ene-VPA, has antiepileptic properties. Another metabolite, 2-n-propyl-4-pentenoic acid (4-ene-VPA), has been proposed as a key hepatotoxic metabolite. The half-life of valproate in adults is 12 to 16 hours. In epileptic patients receiving polytherapy, the half-life is shorter, approximately 9 hours or less in school-age children and young adolescents. Elimination half-lives of valproate are longer in neonates and generally shorter during middle and late infancy. Because hepatic clearance is reduced, the drug's half-life in geriatric patients is approximately 15 hours. Also, because of lower albumin concentrations, the free fraction may be higher in this group.

Dosage and Administration

Oral: Adults, initially 5 to 15 mg/kg/day; usual maintenance dose, 15 to 25 mg/kg/day.

When used with other antiepileptic drugs, the initial dose is 10 to 30 mg/kg/day, and the usual maintenance dose is 30 to 60 mg/kg/day.

Children 1 to 12 years, initially, 10 to 30 mg/kg/day; maintenance dose 20 to 30 mg/kg/day. When used with other antiepileptic drugs that induce hepatic metabolism, the initial dose is 15 to 45 mg/kg/day and the usual maintenance dose is 30 to 100 mg/kg/day. Depakote® Sprinkle may be preferable for use in children and elderly patients because it is more palatable than the syrup, can be sprinkled over food, and is slowly absorbed, which may reduce fluctuations in concentrations.

Depakene® Syrup may be given by nasogastric tube.

Intravenous: A parenteral preparation of valproic acid for intravenous but not intramuscular replacement therapy is now available (Depacon®).

Rectal: Depokene® Syrup may be used rectally.

Valproic Acid:

Generic: capsules 250 mg
Depakene® (Abbott), capsules 250 mg; syrup 250 mg/5 mL
Divalproex Sodium:
Depakote® (Abbott), tablets (delayed-release) 125, 250, and 500 mg.
Depakote® Sprinkle (Abbott), capsules 125 mg.

Adverse Reactions and Precautions

The incidence of gastrointestinal disturbances (nausea, vomiting, anorexia, heartburn) ranges from 6% to 45%. Symptoms are transient and rarely require drug withdrawal. Gastrointenstinal discomfort may be diminished by administering the delayed-release preparation (Depakote® or Depakote® Sprinkle). Diarrhea, abdominal cramps, and constipation are reported occasionally. Increased appetite with weight gain is common and may be controlled by diet, but in some cases, excessive weight gain may require withdrawal of valproate.

Hand tremor, similar to benign essential tremor, is the most common neurologic side effect and occasionally is severe enough to interfere with writing. Tremor occurs more frequently with high doses and may improve with a reduction in dosage.

Sedation and drowsiness develop infrequently in patients receiving valproate alone. Conversely, central nervous system stimulation and excitement have been observed, and aggressiveness and hyperactivity are sometimes noted in children. Ataxia, headache, and stupor have been reported rarely.

Alopecia, thinning, or changes in hair texture occur in some patients, but these effects usually are temporary and do not require the withdrawal of the drug. Rash occurs rarely.

Valproate inhibits the secondary phase of platelet aggregation, but this is usually not clinically significant. However, patients should not receive other drugs that affect coagulation, including aspirin. Thrombocytopenia has been observed, but its incidence is not known. Rarely, hematomas, epistaxis, and increased bleeding after surgery have been reported and platelet function should be monitored before surgery.

A few cases of severe or fatal pancreatitis have been reported. This complication is accompanied by severe abdominal pain, vomiting, and elevated amylase.

Transient elevations of liver transaminases (eg, aspartate aminotransferase [AST]) are common. The elevations usually are not related to serious liver dysfunction, and levels often return to normal with or without dosage adjustment. However, fatal hepatotoxicity has occurred during valproate therapy. Prodromal illness characterized by muscle weakness, lethargy, anorexia, and vomiting is often present. Hepatotoxicity usually develops after an average of 2 months (range, 3 days to 6 months) of therapy (see Chapter 9).

Since 1984, hepatic fatalities associated with the use of valproate have decreased. During 1985 and 1986, five fatalities (none in individuals over 10 years of age) among 198,000 patients were reported (incidence, 1:49,000). This can be attributed to a change in the prescribing patterns for valproate, including increased use of monotherapy and decreased use in high-risk patients.[17]

Guidelines for valproate recommended by the American Academy of Pediatrics and others include:

(1) Avoid administering valproate as polytherapy in children under 3 years of age unless monotherapy has failed to control seizures.

(2) Use other effective therapy initially when possible (eg, in absence and febrile seizures), although valproate is effective in many of these and other types of seizures.

(3) Avoid administering valproate to patients with preexisting hepatic disease or with family history of childhood hepatic disease or to critically ill children and children receiving other medication that affects coagulation.

(4) Assess liver function before therapy, 3 to 5 weeks after initiation of treatment, approximately monthly during the first 6 months of use, and periodically thereafter.

(5) Instruct patients and their parents to report symptoms, such as loss of appetite, lethargy, nausea, vomiting, abdominal pain, jaundice, edema, easy bruising, and loss of seizure control, because laboratory monitoring alone may be inadequate to diagnose valproate-induced hepatotoxicity. However, if laboratory tests indicate clinically important hepatic dysfunction, discontinuation of the drug should be considered.

(6) Maintain dosage at the lowest amount that produces optimal seizure control. Routine monitoring of liver function

does not always detect hepatotoxicity of rapid onset, since it may not be preceded by elevation of AST.

Valproate therapy commonly produces reversible hyperammonemia, but there does not appear to be any clinical significance to this reaction in the absence of liver dysfunction.

Drug Interactions

Valproate inhibits phenobarbital metabolism and the plasma phenobarbital concentration may increase by 25% to 68% when valproate is added.[18] This can cause marked sedation or intoxication attributable to phenobarbital. Therefore, a 30% to 75% reduction in phenobarbital dosage is required when valproate is added to the regimen, and 2 to 3 weeks must elapse before a new steady-state level is achieved.

The interaction between valproate and phenytoin is complex. Valproate displaces phenytoin from plasma albumin, which temporarily increases the ratio of free/bound drug; toxicity may result if phenytoin concentrations were high before administration of valproate. The total phenytoin plasma concentration may decrease by about 30% during the first several weeks of therapy, but usually does not result in recurrence of seizures because the free phenytoin concentration does not change. However, valproate also may inhibit the biotransformation of phenytoin, which, over the next 4 to 16 weeks, produces a gradual return of total phenytoin plasma concentrations to previous values. Measurement of unbound phenytoin concentration may be useful as a means of explaining the onset of central nervous system toxicity when the total plasma phenytoin concentration is within the therapeutic range. Valproate inhibits the metabolism of carbamazepine 10,11-epoxide and of lamotrigine.

Other interactions are detailed in Table 4.

Clonazepam: Actions and Uses

Clonazepam (Klonopin®) may be useful alone or in combination with other drugs to control myoclonic or atonic seizures and photosensitive epilepsy. In patients with juvenile myoclonic epilepsy, clonazepam may help control myoclonic jerks but it has not been shown to be useful for the treatment of generalized tonic-clonic seizures.[19]

Pharmacokinetics

Clonazepam is well absorbed; peak plasma concentrations occur 1 to 4 hours after oral administration. It is almost completely biotransformed to inactive metabolites. The reported half-life ranges are similar for adults (19 to 50 hours) and children (22 to 33 hours).

Dosage and Administration

Oral: Adults, initially 1.5 mg daily in three divided doses, increased by 0.5 to 1 mg every third day until seizures are adequately controlled or until adverse effects occur.

Children, doses of 0.5 mg should be used initially.

Doses for the elderly have not been well established.

Klonopin® (Roche), tablets 0.5, 1, and 2 mg.

Adverse Reactions and Precautions

The most common adverse effects of clonazepam involve the central nervous system. Approximately one half of patients experience drowsiness, about one third ataxia, and up to one quarter personality changes. The sedation may be minimized by initiating therapy with a small dose and increasing the amount gradually.

Drug Interactions

Interactions between clonazepam and other antiepileptic drugs usually are not significant.

Diazepam: Actions and Uses

Intravenous diazepam (Valium®) is effective in continuous tonic-clonic status epilepticus. Its duration of action is short because of its rapid redistribution from the brain. A loading dose of intravenous phenytoin sodium should be given concomitantly or immediately after control of seizures is achieved with diazepam to maintain antiepileptic activity. Maintenance therapy with oral diazepam is not useful in treating epilepsy.

Rectal administration of the parenteral solution of diazepam is effective for the short-term prophylaxis of febrile seizures and treatment of acute repetitive seizures.[20]

Pharmacokinetics

Diazepam's onset of action is almost immediate after intravenous administration. The rectal solution reaches peak concentrations in 5 minutes. The volume of distribution is reported to be 0.95 to 2 L/kg. The half-lives of diazepam and its active derivative, desmethyldiazepam, are 27 to 37, and 50 to 100 hours, respectively; however, rapid redistribution from the brain occurs within 30 minutes after injection.

Dosage and Administration

Intravenous: Adults, 5 to 10 mg initially; then as needed to control seizures.

Intravenous: Children, 0.5 mg, followed by 0.25 mg/kg as needed.

Intravenous: Elderly, 5 mg cautiously, with subsequent doses based on the patient's response.

Rectally: Children, 0.5 to 0.8 mg for children under 3 years of age; 0.6 to 0.9 mg for children over 3 years of age.

Generic: solution 5 mg/mL in 1-mL, 2-mL, and 10-mL containers.

Valium® (Roche), solution 5 mg/mL in 2-mL and 10-mL containers.

Rectal Diastat® (Elan), rectal delivery system, 2.5 mg, 5 mg, and 10 mg for children, and 10 mg, 15 mg, and 20 mg for adults.

Adverse Reactions and Precautions

When diazepam is administered parenterally for the treatment of status epilepticus, the patient must be observed for signs of respiratory and central nervous system depression and hypotension. This is especially true when diazepam is administered with phenobarbital.

Ethosuximide: Actions and Uses

Ethosuximide (Zarontin®) is the drug of choice for absence seizures unaccompanied by other types of seizures. Ethosuximide also may be effective in myoclonic seizures and akinetic epilepsy, but it is generally ineffective in complex partial or generalized tonic-clonic seizures.

Pharmacokinetics

Ethosuximide is well absorbed orally, and the peak plasma concentration occurs in 1 to 4 hours. It is minimally bound to plasma protein and eliminated primarily via hepatic metabolism, with 10% to 20% of the administered dose excreted unchanged in the urine. The half-life is variable but averages 52 to 56 hours in adults and 32 to 41 hours in children. Control of absence seizures usually is achieved with plasma concentrations of 40 to 100 mg/L.

Dosage and Administration

Oral: Adults and children over 6 years of age, initially 500 mg daily, increased if necessary by 250 mg every 4 to 7 days until seizures are controlled or until untoward effects develop. The daily maintenance dose is usually 15 to 40 mg/kg.

Children 3 to 6 years of age, initially 250 mg daily with incremental increases in dosage, as for older patients. The daily maintenance dose is usually 15 to 40 mg/kg.

Zarontin® (Parke-Davis), capsules 250 mg; syrup 250 mg/5 mL.

Adverse Reactions and Precautions

The most common adverse reactions to ethosuximide are gastrointestinal disturbances (eg, nausea, vomiting).

Drug Interactions

Ethosuximide does not consistently alter the plasma concentration of other antiepileptic drugs.

Phenobarbital: Actions and Uses

Phenobarbital (phenobarbital sodium), a long-acting barbiturate, is effective in generalized tonic-clonic and simple partial seizures. Phenobarbital frequently is used to treat neonatal seizures and may be the initial drug employed in young children. However, because of increasing concern about adverse neuropsychologic reactions to sedative/hypnotic antiepileptic drugs, many clinicians prefer less sedating drugs.

Pharmacokinetics

Phenobarbital is almost completely absorbed orally, but 1 to 6 hours may be necessary to achieve peak plasma concentrations. The drug also is well absorbed after intramuscular injection. The average plasma half-life is 3 days in children and 4 days in adults; consequently, 3 or more weeks may be required to attain steady-state plasma concentrations. Plasma concentrations of 15 to 40 mg/L are usually optimal for the control of epilepsy.

Dosage and Administration

Oral: Adults, 120 to 250 mg; alternatively, 2 to 3 mg/kg/day. The elderly may need lower doses. Children, 30 to 100 mg daily; these amounts are taken at bedtime. Administration more than once a day is unnecessary.

Parenteral: Both intramuscular and intravenous administration are well tolerated. It may be given by nasogastric tube.

Generic: elixir 15 and 20 mg/mL; tablets 8, 15, 30, 60, and 100 mg; solution.

Adverse Reactions and Precautions

Phenobarbital is associated with significant behavioral and subtle cognitive effects. Drowsiness is the most common adverse reaction, although tolerance usually develops and a significant percentage of patients continue to experience sedation. Furthermore, phenobarbital may affect memory, perceptual motor performance, and tasks requiring sustained performance. Phenobarbital markedly influences behavior; it can provoke irritability and exacerbate existing behavioral problems, particularly hyperkinesia.

A substantial number of adults who take phenobarbital develop depression. An occasional patient may become excitable; children and the elderly are most susceptible. Phenobarbital must be used cautiously in the elderly because of its propensity to cause sedation, depression, and mental slowing. These side effects may either exacerbate existing symptoms of declining brain function or may be confused for the onset of dementia. Abrupt termination of therapy may exacerbate seizures, but drug dependence is unlikely with usual antiepileptic doses. Skin eruptions are uncommon.

Drug Interactions

Phenobarbital both induces hepatic enzymes and competitively inhibits drug biotransformation. Thus, mutual enzyme induction or inhibition in patients treated with phenobarbital and phenytoin may result in an increase, decrease, or no change in the plasma concentration of one or both of the drugs.

Because it induces hepatic enzymes, phenobarbital may enhance the hepatic clearance and decrease the clinical effectiveness of many other drugs (Table 4).

Primidone: Actions and Uses

Primidone (Mysoline®) is a deoxybarbiturate closely related chemically to the barbiturates. It is converted to two active metabolites, phenobarbital and phenylethylmalonamide (PEMA). Primidone is used principally in generalized tonic-clonic and complex and simple partial seizures. It is as effective as carbamazepine or phenytoin in controlling partial or generalized tonic-clonic seizures, although its greater incidence of adverse reactions limits patient acceptance.[5]

Pharmacokinetics

Primidone is rapidly and completely absorbed after oral administration; peak plasma concentrations are attained in an average of 4 hours, but there is wide interpatient variation. Because phenobarbital is the major active metabolite of primidone, its plasma concentrations should be measured and are usually 2 to 3 times higher than that of primidone.

Dosage and Administration

Oral: Adults and older children, initially 125 mg at bedtime for 3 days, with the dose increased by 125 mg every 3 days until a maintenance dose of 250 mg 3 times a day is established on the 10th day.

Children under 8 years of age, initially one half of the adult dosage. For maintenance, 125 mg to 250 mg is given 3 times a day.

Generic: tablets 250 mg

Mysoline® (Elan), suspension 250 mg/5 mL; tablets 50 and 250 mg.

Adverse Reactions and Precautions

Similar to phenobarbital.

Acetazolamide: Action and Uses

Acetazolamide (Ak-Zol®, Diamox®), a carbonic anhydrase inhibitor, has been used in absence, generalized tonic-clonic, and partial seizures. It is most often administered as an adjunct to other drugs, but its usefulness is limited by the rapid development of tolerance in some patients. Acetazolamide is most widely used intermittently in women whose seizure frequency increases with menstruation.

Dosage and Administration

Oral: Adults and children, 8 to 30 mg/kg daily in divided doses (range, 250 mg to 1 g daily).

Generic: tablets 250 mg

Ak-Zol® (Akorn), tablets 250 mg.

Newer Antiepileptic Drugs

Eight drugs have been approved since 1993 (Table 2), while a number of other AEDs are still in clinical trials.

Gabapentin

(Neurontin®, Parke-Davis)

Action and Uses

Gabapentin is a GABA-related amino acid that readily penetrates the blood brain barrier but its specific mechanism of action is not yet clear. Several clinical studies have evaluated the safety and efficacy of gabapentin.[21,22] In a double-blind, parallel design study, 127 patients with refractory partial epilepsy were randomized to placebo or to 1200 mg/day of gabapentin. Twenty-six percent of the treated patients had a reduction in seizure frequency greater than 50%, versus 10% of the placebo-treated patients (p=0.042). In the U.S. study, 306 patients with refractory partial epilepsy received doses of 600, 1200, or 1800 mg/day.[22] A dose-related decrease in seizures was observed at the higher doses. In clinical use, doses of 2400 to 6000 mg/day have been used and are well tolerated.

Long-term studies of gabapentin have shown that it is well tolerated and does not lose its efficacy over time.[23,24] More than 400,000 patients have been treated with gabapentin with no major adverse reactions linked to this drug. The FDA approved gabapentin for use in adults as an add-on therapy for partial and secondarily generalized seizures. Monotherapy studies have been completed and approval is pending. Its major difference from other antiepileptic medications is its lack of interactions with other drugs. The use of gabapentin in children with epilepsy has been studied and been shown to be well tolerated. Since its introduction for use in epilepsy, gabapentin has been shown to be effective in certain chronic pain syndromes but this is not an approved FDA indication.

The age group in which gabapentin may be most useful is the elderly. These patients are most likely to be on many other drugs, and gabapentin may be the best tolerated and least problematic. In clinical practice, blood levels of 2 to 20 mg/L have been found to be effective.

Pharmacokinetics

The oral bioavailability of gabapentin is approximately 60% in humans. The time to maximum concentration is 2 to 4 hours after a dose is taken. Gabapentin does not bind to human plasma proteins. After intravenous administration, its terminal elimination half-life is approximately 5 hours.[24,25] The renal clearance of gabapentin equals the total clearance in normal volunteers and is 120 to 130 mL/min. No metabolite has been detected in human beings. After single doses, a linear correlation has been demonstrated between dose and the 2-hour plasma concentration in patients on gabapentin monotherapy.[24,25]

Doses

The initital dose of gabapentin in adults is 900 mg/day in divided doses. It can be rapidly titrated, 300 mg on day one, 300 mg b.i.d. day two, and then 300 mg t.i.d. Doses of 6000 mg/day have been well tolerated in adults.

Adverse Reactions and Precautions

The most common side effects from gabapentin are mild fatigue and dizziness.[25] Other side effects have been nystagmus, hypotension, diarrhea, muscle weakness, dry mouth, sleep disturbances, slurred speech, decreased alertness, tremor, rash, and nausea. There have been no changes in the hematologic and biochemical parameters.[21]

Gabapentin in very large doses appears to have little toxicity; one patient took 48 g in an attempted suicide. Even though blood levels were initltially over 60 mg/mL, clearance was rapid and she experienced minimal symptoms.[26]

Drug Interactions

The major feature of gabapentin is its lack of interaction with other drugs.[26] Unlike the other antiepileptic medications, gabapentin is not metabolized by the liver. It is almost completely eliminated by renal excretion of the parent compound. Thus, it does not affect the concentrations of the other antiepileptic drugs,[27] and may have few interactions with other drugs as well. It is especially useful in patients who are receiving many other medications, such as the elderly.

Gabapentin: Neurontin® gelatin capsules, 100, 300, 400 mg, and tablets 600, 800 mg.

Lamotrigine

(Lamictal®, Glaxo Wellcome)

Action and Uses

In animal studies it appears that lamotrigine may act at voltage-sensitive sodium channels to stabilize neuronal membranes and inhibit transmitter release, primarily glutamate.[28]

Clinical studies have demonstrated lamotrigine to be effective in adults with partial and generalized seizures.[29-32] It was approved for use in December 1994 for adults with complex partial seizures and secondarily generalized seizures. The use of lamotrigine in children with epilepsy has been studied.

Pharmacokinetics

Lamotrigine is rapidly absorbed after oral dosing and is 55% protein bound.[29] Lamotrigine is extensively metabolized and excreted predominantly as a glucuronide. In normal volunteers, the mean terminal elimination half-life is 24 hours. Patients receiving either phenytoin or carbamazepine were found to have a shorter half-life, 15 hours (range 7.8 to 33 hours). In patients receiving valproate, the lamotrigine half-life was 59 hours (range 30 to 89 hours). In clinical practice, effective serum concentrations of lamotrigine vary from 2 to 20 mg/L.

Doses

Doses of 75 to 600 mg/day have been used in studies of adults with epilepsy but doses of up to 1,600 mg may be needed in polytherapy. The initial doses of lamotrigine must be adjusted to concomitant medications. If the patient is on enzyme-inducing antiepileptic drugs but not valproate, the dose should be 50 mg/day for 2 weeks, then 100 mg for the next two weeks, and then the dose can be increased by 100 mg each week to a dose of 300 to 500 mg/day. If the patient is on valproate, the initial dose should be 25 mg every other day for two weeks, then 25 mg/day for the next two weeks, then increased by 25 to 50 mg every week or two to a dose of 100 to 150 mg/day.

Adverse Reactions

The most frequently reported side effects of lamotrigine have been diplopia, drowsiness, ataxia, and headache.[30] A higher incidence of skin rash has been observed in patients receiving concomitant valproic acid. In children, a high rate of serious skin rashes, including Stevens-Johnson syndrome, has occurred. In March 1997, the manufacturer added a warning that the rate of serious rash may occur in 1:50 to 1:100 children. Therefore, lamotrigine must be used cautiously in children. Slow titration appears to lessen the incidence of skin rashes. Clinical experience has shown that serum concentrations between 2.0 and 20.0 mg/L have been effective and tolerated.

Drug Interactions

Lamotrigine does not appear to affect the concentrations of other antiepileptic drugs. However, other drugs affect lamotrigine. Valproate causes a marked prolongation of lamotrigine half-life, to almost double or triple its half-life when used alone. Phenytoin and carbamazepine significantly shorten lamotrigine's half-life.

Lamotrigine: Lamictal® tablets, 25, 100, 150, 200 mg.

Felbamate

(Felbatol®, Wallace Laboratories)

Actions and Uses

Felbamate appears to increase seizure threshold.[33] Its effectiveness was demonstrated in a number of studies in adults with partial and generalized seizures.[34,35] Felbamate has also been shown to reduce atonic seizures and to improve the global assessment scores in children with Lennox-Gastaut syndrome.[36] In July 1993, the FDA granted approval of felbamate for both add-on therapy and as monotherapy in adults with partial seizures with or without generalization and in children with partial and generalized seizures associated with the Lennox-Gastaut syndrome. However, a strong warning was added in September, 1994, because of reports of aplastic anemia and hepatitis. Physicians and patients must read the most current 'black box' warning in the package insert before using this drug. Because of its association with aplastic anemia, felbamate should be reserved for those patients for whom there is no other effective alternative treatment.

Pharmacokinetics

The elimination half-life of felbamate is approximately 15 to 20 hours and its pharmacokinetics appear to be linear. Time to maximum concentration occurs 1 to 4 hours after a dose is administered. Plasma protein binding is not clinically significant.

Doses

In adults, doses during clinical trials have ranged from 1800 to 4800 mg/day. In children, doses of 15 to 45 mg/kg have been used. With monotherapy, larger doses are tolerated.

Adverse Reactions and Toxicity

Animal studies and clinical trials showed no effect of felbamate on hematologic or hepatic function. No major adverse events were noted during the clinical trials involving more than 2,000 patients. However, after use exceeded 100,000 patients, 32 cases of aplastic anemia and 10 cases of hepatitis were reported. Monitoring of laboratory parameters monthly during the first year and then quarterly is recommended for those patients needing felbamate for refractory epilepsy. Side effects include insomnia, weight loss, nausea, decreased appetite, dizziness, fatigue, ataxia, and lethargy. There were substantially higher rates of side effects in persons receiving other antiepileptic medications, and conversion to monotherapy often reduced side effects.

Drug Interactions

Felbamate has significant interactions with phenytoin, carbamazepine, and valproate. The concentrations of phenytoin and valproate increase with felbamate. Therefore, when felbamate is initiated, the doses of these other agents should be decreased by 20% to 40% or more. On the other hand, carbamazepine concentrations decrease by about 20% when felbamate is added to therapy. The concentrations of felbamate are lowered by the concomitant use of other antiepileptic drugs, especially those that induce hepatic enzymes.

Felbamate: Felbatol® tablets, 400 mg, 600 mg; oral suspension 600 mg/5 mL.

Topiramate

(Topamax®, Ortho-McNeil Pharmaceutical)

Action and Uses

Topiramate is a sulfamate-substituted monosaccharide that appears to have at least three distinct mechanisms of action in the central nervous system.[38] It appears to block repetitive firing of the sodium channel, to increase the frequency of γ-aminobutyrate (GABA) activation at GABA$_A$ receptors, and to antagonize the ability of the excitatory amino acid kainate to activate the kainate/AMPA receptor. Therefore, it has a unique profile of mechanisms covering a wide range of inhibitory and excitatory actions.

Pharmacokinetics

Absorption is rapid, with peak plasma concentrations occurring in 2 hours; bioavailability is approximately 80%, and its half-life is 21 hours. It is not extensively metabolized, with approximately 70% excreted unchanged in the urine.[39]

Doses

In clinical trials of doses of 200, 400, 600, and 1,000 mg per day, there did not appear to be an increase of efficacy at the higher doses, but side effects were more common.[40] The recommended daily dose for adults is 400 mg in two divided doses. Therapy should be initiated at 25 mg/day to 50 mg/day and increased by 25-mg to 50-mg increments.

Adverse Reactions and Toxicity

The most common adverse reactions are somnolence, dizziness, ataxia, speech disorders, psychomotor slowing, and paresthesias. Significant kidney stones occurred in approximately 1.5% of patients during clinical trials, an incidence 2 to 4 times that expected in a similar, untreated population.

Drug Interactions

Topiramate does not appear to affect levels of other drugs. However, phenytoin and carbamazepine decrease topiramate concentrations by 48% and 40%, respectively.

Topiramate: Topamax® tablets, 25, 100, 200 mg.

Tiagabine

(Gabitril®, Abbott Laboratories)

Action and Uses

Tiagabine is a blocker of GABA reuptake, thus increasing GABA concentrations in the synaptic cleft. Its major effect is to enhance the activity of GABA, the major neuroinhibitory transmitter in the central nervous system.[41] It has been found effective for the treatment of partial seizures.[42] It is approved for use as adjunctive therapy in adults and children 12 years and older in the treatment of partial seizures.

Pharmacokinetics

Absorption is rapid, with peak concentrations occurring approximately 45 min after an oral dose. Its half-life is 7 to 9 hours in volunteers, but may be 4 to 7 hours in patients receiving drugs that induce hepatic enzymes.[43] It is extensively metabolized by the CYP 3A isoform subfamily of cytochrome P-450, with only 2% of the dose excreted unchanged. Tiagabine is highly (96%) protein bound, mostly to serum albumin and α1-acid glycoprotein.

Doses

In adults, tiagabine should be initiated at 4 mg once a day, increased by 4 to 8 mg at weekly intervals, up to 56 mg per day. Doses of 120 mg have been used in some patients, especially those who are receiving other drugs that stimulate hepatic metabolism.

Adverse Reactions and Toxicity

The most common adverse events in placebo-controlled trials were referable to the CNS and consisted of somnolence, dizziness, and difficulty with concentration.[44] No systematic abnormalities on routine laboratory tests were noted during the studies, and no specific recommendations regarding routine monitoring have been made. Patients with a history of spike-wave abnormalities on EEG may have an exacerbation as well as clinical symptoms of lethargy or poor responsiveness.

Drug Interactions

Tiagabine has been shown not to have an effect on most drugs, including oral contraceptives. However, drugs that induce hepatic metabolism, especially phenytoin, phenobarbital, and carbamazepine, significantly increase the metabolism of tiagabine and lead to the need for higher doses.

Tiagabine: 4-mg, 12-mg, 16-mg, and 20-mg tablets.

Levetiracetam

(Keppra®, UCB Pharma)

Actions and Uses

Levetiracetam is indicated for use as adjunctive treatment of partial onset seizures in adults with epilepsy. Its precise mechanism of action is unknown, but it does not act by any known mechanisms. It was not active in earlier models of animal experiments of epileptic seizures, but was potent in newer models. Thus, its full clinical spectrum remains to be explored.[45]

Pharmacokinetics

Levetiracetam is rapidly absorbed (peak absorption 1 hour after administration) and its oral bioavailability is close to 100%. It is very water soluble, and its volume of distribution is similar to that of intracellular and extracellular water. Protein binding is less than 10%. It passes the blood-brain barrier rapidly and is bound to a stereoselective binding site in synaptic membranes. Levetiracetam is mostly excreted unchanged in the urine. Less than 25% is metabolized by hydrolysis and is not dependent on any of the cytochrome P-450 isoenzymes. Its plasma half-life in adults is 6 to 8 hours, but its pharmacokinetic half-life is longer.

Dosage and Administration

Initial adult doses of levetiracetam are 500 mg b.i.d. Clinical studies have shown 1,000 mg/day to be effective. Doses may be increased in increments of 1,000 mg/day. The maximum recommended dose is 3,000 mg/day. Pediatric doses appear to be in the range of 20 to 40 mg/kg/day. In elderly patients and others with decreased renal function, doses may need to be reduced.

Levetiracetam

Generic: none
Keppra®: tablets 250 mg, 500 mg, 750 mg

Adverse Reactions and Precautions

In placebo-controlled studies, dizziness, somnolence, and asthenia were the most commonly reported side effects. No serious idiosyncratic adverse events have been noted.

Drug Interactions

Pharmacokinetic interactions between levetiracetam and phenytoin, warfarin, digoxin, and oral contraceptives have been excluded by clinical studies because of its lack of protein-binding and independence of the P-450 pathways. Other drug interactions are unlikely.

Oxcarbazepine

Actions and Uses

Oxcarbazepine (Trileptal®) is recommended as adjunctive treatment in partial seizures in adults and as adjunctive treatment for partial seizures in children ages 4 to 16.[46]

Pharmacokinetics

Oxcarbazepine is inactive but is metabolized into 10-monohydroxy oxcarbazepine (MHD). Oxcarbazepine is completely absorbed with an average Tmax of 4.5 hour. It then has a plasma half-life of approximately 2 hours, while MHD has a half-life of approximately 9 hours. Approximately 70% of oxcarbazepine is converted to MHD, the rest to inactive metabolites. Approximately 40% is protein bound.

Dosage and Administration

As monotherapy, treatment with oxcarbazepine should be initiated with a dose of 300 mg b.i.d. in adults, and increased by 300 mg every third day to a dose of 1,200 mg/day. As adjunctive therapy, treatment can be initiated at 300 mg b.i.d. and increased as needed. To convert to monotherapy, other AEDs can then be decreased over 3 to 6 weeks, or longer, as clinically indicated. In general, 300 mg of oxcarbazepine is equivalent to 200 mg of carbamazepine.

For children, initial doses should be 8 to 10 mg/kg/day b.i.d. Doses can be increased to 20 to 40 mg/kg/day. Children under 8 years of age may need doses 30% to 40% greater.

Oxcarbazepine

Generic: none
Trileptal®: tablets 150 mg, 300 mg, 600 mg

Adverse Reactions and Precautions

Like carbamazepine, oxcarbazepine may be associated with hyponatremia. In placebo-controlled studies, 38 of 1,524 (2.5%) patients treated with oxcarbazepine had serum sodium concentrations of less than 125 mmol/L compared to none treated with placebo. In addition, 25% to 30% of patients who had a hypersensitivity reaction to carbamazepine developed a similar reaction to oxcarbazepine. Most common side effects are related to the central nervous system, and include dizziness, somnolence, diplopia, fatigue, and ataxia.

Drug Interactions

Oxcarbazepine can inhibit CYP 2C19 and induce CYP 3A4/5. Thus, oxcarbazepine may increase phenytoin concentrations (metabolized by CYP 2C19) by as much as 40%. By inducing CYP 3A, hormonal contraceptives may be rendered less effective.

Zonisamide

Action and Uses

Zonisamide (Zonegran®) is recommended as adjunctive treatment for partial seizures in adults and children (over 12 years of age). It has been available in Japan for more than 10 years, and the experience there, as well as from compassionate use, suggests it may be very effective for certain myoclonic syndromes.[47,48]

Pharmacokinetics

Zonisamide is rapidly absorbed with a Tmax of 2 to 3 hours and has a long half-life. In human volunteers, its half-life is more than 60 hours, but this is shortened to about 30 hours when used with drugs that induce hepatic metabolism. Twice-a-day dosing is appropriate. It is predominantly metabolized by the liver, but a significant amount is excreted in the urine as unchanged drug. Protein binding is low.

Dosage and Administration

Zonisamide can be started as 100 mg to 200 mg/day in adults, and 2 to 4 mg/kg/day in children. Steady state is reached in 7 to 10 days, and doses can be increased at 2-week intervals. Maintenance doses are 400 to 600 mg/day in adults and 4 to 8 mg/kg/day in children.

Zonisamide

Generic: none
Zonegran®: tablets 100 mg

Adverse Reactions and Precautions

The most serious adverse event is the development of significant renal calculi in approximately 1.5% of persons in clinical trials in the United States. Interestingly, renal calculi have not been observed in Japan. Other adverse effects include somnolence, ataxia, anorexia, confusion, fatigue, and dizziness.

Drug Interactions

Zonisamide does not induce hepatic enzymes and thus does not appear to affect the metabolism of other drugs. However, in persons receiving either phenytoin or carbamazepine, the half-life of zonisamide was observed to be approximately 30 hours.[49] On the other hand, lamotrigene may inhibit the clearance of zonisamide.

References

1. Federal Food, Drug, and Cosmetic Act of 1938, Public Law 717, 75th Congress.

2. Merritt HH, Putnam TJ: Sodium diphenylhydantoinate in the treatment of convulsive disorders. *JAMA* 1938;111:1068-1073.

3. Michalets EL: Update: clinically significant cytochrome P-450 drug interactions. *Pharmacotherapy* 1998;18(1):84-112.

4. Snead OC III, Hosey LC: Exacerbation of seizures in children by carbamazepine. *N Engl J Med* 1985;313:916-921.

5. Mattson RH, et al: Comparison of carbamazepine, phenobarbital, phenytoin, and primidone in partial and secondarily generalized tonic-clonic seizures. *N Engl J Med* 1985;313:145-151.

6. Bourgeois BFD, Wad NL: Individualized and combined antiepileptic and neurotoxic activity of carbamazepine and carbamazepine-10,11-epoxide in mice. *J Pharmacol Exp Ther* 1984;231:411-415.

7. Porter RJ: How to initiate and maintain carbamazepine therapy in children and adults. *Epilepsia* 1987;28(suppl 3):S59-S63.

8. Pellock JM: Carbamazepine side effects in children and adults. *Epilepsia* 1987; 28(suppl 3):S64-S70.

9. Lahr MB: Hyponatremia during carbamazepine therapy. *Clin Pharmacol Ther* 1985; 37:693-696.

10. Wagner JG: New and simple method to predict dosage of drugs obeying simple Michaelis-Menten elimination kinetics and to distinguish such kinetics from simple first order and from parallel Michaelis-Menten and first order kinetics. *Ther Drug Monit* 1985;7:377-386.

11. Nuwer MR, Browne TR, Dodson WE, et al: Generic substitutions for antiepileptic drugs. *Neurology* 1990;40:1647-1651.

12. Leppik IE, Fisher J, Kriel R, et al: Altered phenytoin clearance during febrile illness. *Neurology* 1986;36:1367-1370.

13. Haley CJ, Nelson J: Phenytoin-enteral feeding interaction. *Ann Pharmacother* 1989;23:796-798.

14. Leppik IE, Boucher BA, Wilder BJ, et al: Pharmacokinetics and safety of a phenytoin prodrug given IV or IM in patients. *Neurology* 1990;40:456-460.

15. Leppik IE, Lapora J, Lowenson R, et al: Seasonal incidence of phenytoin allergy unrelated to plasma levels. *Arch Neurol* 1985;42:120-122.

16. Mattson RH, Cramer JA, Collins JF, et al: Valproate vs carbamazepine for seizures, a comparison of valproate with carbamazepine for the treatment of complex partial seizures and secondarily generalized tonic-clonic seizures in adults. *N Engl J Med* 1992;327(11):765.

17. Dreifuss FE, Santilli N, Langer DH, et al: Valproic acid hepatic fatalities: a retrospective review. *Neurology* 1987;37:379-385.

18. Richens A, Ahmad S: Controlled trial of sodium valproate in severe epilepsy. *Br Med J* 1975;4:255-256.

19. Obeid T, Panayiotopoulos CP: Clonazepam in juvenile myoclonic epilepsy. *Epilepsia* 1989;30:603-606.

20. Dreifuss FE, Rosman NP, Cloyd JC, et al: A comparison of rectal diazepam gel and placebo for acute repetitive seizures. *N Engl J Med* 1998;338:1869-1875.

21. Bartoszyk GD, Meyerson N. Reimann W, et al: Gabapentin. In: Meldrum BS, Porter RJ, eds. *New Anticonvulsant Drugs*. London, John Libbey, 1986, pp 147-163.

22. Leiderman DB: Gabapentin as add-on therapy for refractory partial epilepsy: Results of five placebo-controlled trials. *Epilepsia* 1994;35 (suppl 5):S74-S76.

23. Sivenius J, Ylinen A, Kalviainen R, et al: Long-term study with gabapentin in patients with epileptic seizures. *Arch Neurol* 1994; 51(10):1047-1050.

24. The U.S. Gabapentin Study Group: The long-term safety and efficacy of gabapentin (Neurontin) as add-on therapy in partial epilepsy. *Epilepsy Res* 1994;18(1):67-73.

25. Schmidt D: Potential antiepileptic drugs: Gabapentin. In: Levy R, Mattson R, Meldrum B, et al, eds. *Antiepileptic Drugs*, 3rd ed. New York, Raven Press, 1989, pp 925-935.

26. Fisher JH, Barr AN, Rogers SL, et al: Lack of serious toxicity following gabapentin overdose. *Neurology* 1994;44(5):982-983.

27. Graves NM, Holmes GB, Leppik IE: Pharmacokinetics of gabapentin in patients treated with phenytoin. *Pharmacotherapy* 1989; 9:196.

28. Miller AA, Sawyer DA, Roth B: Lamotrigine. In: Meldrum B, Porter RJ, eds. *New Anticonvulsant Drugs*. London, John Libbey, 1986, pp 165-177.

29. Gram L: Potential antiepileptic drugs: Lamotrigine. In: Levy R, Mattson R, Meldrum B, et al, eds. *Antiepileptic Drugs*, 3rd ed. New York, Raven Press, 1989, pp 947-953.

30. Jawad S, Richens A, Goodwin G, et al: Controlled trial of lamotrigine (Lamictal) for refractory partial seizures. *Epilepsia* 1989;30:356-363.

31. Binnie CD, Beintema CJ, Debets RMC, et al: Seven-day administration of lamotrigine (Lamictal) for refractory partial seizures. *Epilepsia* 1987;1:202-208.

32. Messenheimer J, Ramsey RE, Willmore LJ, et al: Lamotrigine therapy for partial seizures: A multicenter, placebo-controlled, double-blind, cross-over trial. *Epilepsia* 1994;35(1):13-21.

33. Swinyard EA, Sofia RD, Kupferberg HJ: Comparative anticonvulsant activity and neurotoxicity of felbamate and four prototype antiepileptic drugs in mice and rats. *Epilepsia* 1986;27:27-34.

34. Leppik IE, Dreifuss, FE, Pledger GW, et al: Felbamate for partial seizures: Results of a controlled clinical trial. *Neurology* 1991;41:1785-1789.

35. Sachedo R, Kramer LD, Rosenberg A, et al: Felbamate monotherapy: Controlled trial in patients with partial onset seizures. *Ann Neurol* 1992;32:286-292.

36. The Felbamate Study Group in Lennox-Gastaut syndrome. Efficacy of felbamate in childhood epileptic encephalopathy (Lennox-Gastaut syndrome). *N Engl J Med* 1993;328:29-33.

37. Leppik IE, Wolff DL: The place of felbamate in the treatment of epilepsy. *CNS Drugs* 1995;4:294-301.

38. Bialer M, Johannessen SI, Kupferberg HJ, et al: Progress report on new antiepileptic drugs: a summary of the Third Eilat Conference. *Epilepsy Res (Netherlands)* 1996;3:299-319.

39. Doose DR, Walker SA, Gisclon LG, et al: Single-dose pharmacokinetics and effect of food on the bioavailability of topiramate, a novel antiepileptic drug. *J Clin Pharmacol* 1996;36(10):884-991.

40. Faught E, Wilder BJ, Ramsey RE, et al: Topiramate placebo-controlled dose-ranging trial in refractory partial epilepsy using 200-, 400-, and 600-mg daily dosages. *Neurology* 1996;46(6):1684-1690.

41. Suzdak PD, Jansen JA: A review of the preclinical pharmacology of tiagabine: a potent and selective anticonvulsant GABA uptake inhibitor. *Epilepsia* 1995;36:612-626.

42. Richens A, Chadwick DW, Duncan JS, et al: Adjunctive treatment of partial seizures with tiagabine: a placebo-controlled trial. *Epilepsy Res* 1995;21:37-42.

43. Brodie MJ: Tiagabine pharmacology in profile. *Epilepsia* 1995;36:S7-S9.

44. Leppik IE: Tiagabine: the safety landscape. *Epilepsia* 1995;36:S10-S13.

45. Bialer M, Johannessen SI, Kupferberg HJ, et al: Progress report on new antiepileptic drugs: a summary of the fourth Eilat conference (EILAT IV). *Epilepsy Res* 1999;34(1):1-41.

46. Schachter SC, Vazquez B, Fisher RS, et al: Oxcarbazepine: double-blind, randomized, placebo-control, monotherapy trial for partial seizures. *Neurology* 1999;52:732-737.

47. Leppik IE: Zonisamide. *Epilepsia* 1999;40(suppl 5):S23-S29.

48. Henry T, Leppik IE, Gumnit RJ, et al: Progressive myoclonus epilepsy treated with zonisamide. *Neurology* 1988;38:928-931.

49. Ojemann LM, Shastri RA, Wilensky AJ, et al: Comparative pharmacokinetics of zonisamide (CI-912) in epileptic patents on carbamazepine or phenytoin monotherapy. *Ther Drug Monit* 1986;8(3):293-296.

Chapter 8

Measuring Antiepileptic Drug Concentrations and Patient Compliance

A ppropriate measurements of AED concentrations can contribute to cost-effective management of epilepsy. Measurement of AED concentrations is essential five times during the course of treatment (Table 1). First, when an AED has been started, it is useful to obtain a measurement to determine the patient's metabolism. For example, most adults given 5 mg/kg/day of phenytoin achieve steady-state concentrations of 10 mg/mL to 15 mg/mL. However, some patients are deficient in parahydroxylase, and may become toxic on this dose; some are rapid metabolizers and attain lower levels. The information obtained from this measurement can guide future adjustments of dose. The second time is when the goal of control has been achieved. This concentration can then be used as the patient's individual therapeutic range, or target value. The third is to measure compliance. This is especially useful at times of license renewal to verify that the patient is continuing to take the medicine as directed. If levels are below the target value, clinicians should be concerned about an increased risk for seizures. The fourth time is when the patient suffers from breakthrough seizures. If the concentration is at the target value, there may have been a change in the person's susceptibility for seizures, either because of an intercurrent illness, or worsening of the epileptic syndrome. On the other hand, if the levels are below the target value, noncompliance, or the addition of another drug that increased clearance, must be suspected. The fifth time to measure levels is when the patient experiences symptoms of toxicity. It is best to get a blood sample when the patient is toxic because, with some of the drugs with short half-lives, levels can fall back to the target value in a few hours.

A number of devices exists for measuring medication concentrations in plasma, serum, saliva, and other biological samples (Figure 1). Gas liquid chromatography was the initial technique.[1] It has been replaced by high-performance

Table 1: AED Monitoring in Patients with Epilepsy*

1. to obtain dose-level information
2. at steady state, good control to get target level
3. to monitor compliance, annually
4. at breakthrough seizure
5. whenever symptoms of toxicity occur

* Trough measurements are primarily useful for pharmacokinetic studies. Levels drawn for target levels and compliance should be obtained at similar times of day, within 1 to 2 hours of each other.

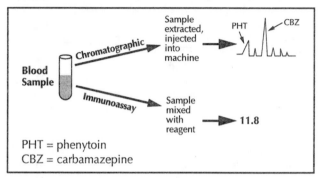

PHT = phenytoin
CBZ = carbamazepine

Figure 1—Two major kinds of systems are used to measure AED concentrations. The chromatographic system produces a graphic output and measures concentrations as peak heights. Most immunoassay systems have internalized a number of steps, with the concentration determined photometrically after various reactions have taken place. The concentration is usually displayed as a number.

liquid chromatography in most laboratories.[2] It can measure a number of AEDs from the same sample.

In the clinical setting, immunoassays are preferred because they require fewer operator skills.[3,4] Other systems are being developed. To be approved by the U.S. Food and Drug Administration, a device for therapeutic drug monitoring must be able to perform with a coefficient of variation (CV) of less than 5%. Although all of these devices meet this standard under strict testing conditions, the potential for error exists in clinical settings. It is reasonable to assume that less than 5%

of the variability in serial AED determinations can be attributed to measurement error if testing is done by a certified laboratory. Most of the variability between serial measurements of AED concentrations over time in a patient can be attributed to pharmacokinetics and compliance.

Pharmacokinetics

A number of pharmacokinetic factors can influence the absorption and elimination of AEDs. For example, changes in product formulation can alter the absorption of phenytoin to the degree that toxic reactions or breakthrough can occur.[5,6] In the case of permissible or mandated generic substitution, product formulations may play a role in creating variable drug concentrations. Alteration of gastric or intestinal absorption by food or other drugs may influence the time or extent of absorption.[7] To a small degree, changes in hepatic or renal blood flow can modify the rate of clearance and affect medication concentrations.[8]

Time of sampling may contribute to variability in AED levels. Phenytoin has a relatively long absorption time (time to maximum concentration of 6 to 12 hours) because of its uptake in the small intestine. Nonlinear kinetics give it an elimination half-life of 18 to 36 hours. Thus, one cycle of absorption and elimination can be on the order of 24 to 46 hours. With more than once-a-day administration, the absorption and elimination phases overlap and the concentration differences are small between peak and trough levels. Carbamazepine and valproate both have shorter absorption times and, during long-term therapy, elimination half-lives of 6 to 14 hours.

The Importance of Compliance

Noncompliance with AEDs is a major factor in the recurrence of seizures in patients with epilepsy. As many as 50% of all patients with epilepsy are noncompliant to a degree that interferes with optimal treatment.[9,10] Studies using electronic monitors to measure compliance indicate that what may appear to be sporadic seizures can be attributed to missed doses of AEDs.[11] Consequently, proper management of epilepsy requires physicians to identify noncompliant patients, determine the causes and extent of the problem, and devise and monitor an appropriate intervention strategy.

Table 2: **Types of Behavior in Noncompliance Medication Ingestion**

- Consistent overcompliance
- Consistent undercompliance
- Irregular
  - irregularly irregular
  - sporadically irregular
  - cyclically irregular

Prescription filling
Medical appointments

Life-style

Sleep patterns
Alcohol use
Psychological stress
Exposure to music, strobe lights
Drug abuse
Adherence to regulations

Intentionality of Compliance

Patient controlled
- Rational
  - pregnant women afraid of teratogenicity
  - compensation-related
- Irrational
  - fear of medicine
  - superstition

Structural

- Memory deficit
- Financial problems

Noncompliant behavior may significantly increase healthcare costs.[12] An increased number of seizures would result in rising fees for ambulance transportation, emergency department visits, and hospitalization, as well as for medical treatment and drugs. In addition, seizures experienced at work or in recreational settings have social costs. Moreover, noncompliant patients run the risk of endangering others, for example, by having seizures while driving or by injuring an unborn child if seizures occur during pregnancy. Status epilepticus may be associated with subtherapeutic AED concentrations, probably from missed doses.[13]

Treatment of epilepsy requires that stable drug concentrations be maintained at the active receptor site at all times. Unlike pain or infections, for which intermittent attainment of analgesic or bactericidal concentrations is acceptable, epilepsy is best controlled when as little variation as possible occurs over time in medication concentrations. One of the most common precipitants of a seizure is a reduction in drug concentrations, either from missed doses[14] or from an illness that increases metabolism and thereby lowers therapeutic levels.[15]

Only a twofold to threefold difference in AEDs separates the lowest effective concentration from toxic levels. For example, the usual effective range for phenytoin is 10 to 20 mg/L; for carbamazepine, 4 to 12 mg/L; and for valproate, 50 to 100 mg/L. These ranges are much narrower than for most other classes of drugs. Although pharmacokinetic factors can influence medication levels, compliance generally determines whether a stable concentration will be maintained.

Defining Compliance

Compliance is a multidimensional variable characterized by type of behavior, extent of compliance, and degree of intention (Table 2). Patient compliance with medication ingestion, which most concerns physicians, generally has three patterns: irregular ingestion, sporadic irregularity, and cyclical irregularity. These may well have different causes. Irregular ingestion is most common. Sporadic irregularity may be event related, ie, stemming from a busy week. Cyclical irregularity may be prompted by specific schedules, such as weekend trips.

Extent of compliance must be viewed as a continuum of behavior, which ranges from the rare patient who takes every prescribed dose precisely as directed, to the consistently noncompliant patient. Most patients fall somewhere between these extremes. Much of the variability in AED concentrations not accounted for by small pharmacokinetically induced fluctuations can be attributed to noncompliance.

There are many ways to assess compliance, but the methods can be divided into two categories: direct or indirect (Table 3). The direct methods involve technologies such as measuring AED levels in blood or using devices that record when patients take their pills. Other studies have used measurements of AED levels in patients' blood to evaluate compliance and identify as noncompliant those whose levels fall

121

Table 3: Methods By Which Compliance Can Be Measured

Direct

- Measurement of isolated AED levels
- Serial measurement of AED levels to determine variability
- Recording pill-taking behavior with electronic devices

Indirect

- Patient interview
- Therapeutic outcome
- Physician's judgment
- Interviews with caregivers
- Pill counts

AED = antiepileptic drug

$$\text{Coefficient of variation } (\%) = \frac{\text{standard deviation} \times 100}{X}$$

X = mean of plasma concentration measurements

Figure 2—Calculating the degree of fluctuation by using the coefficient of variation.

outside the usual therapeutic range. Patients whose levels are within normal range are then considered compliant. This method is simplistic, however, because compliant patients may be receiving doses that are too low for their body weight and, consequently, have levels below normal range.

Indirect assessments rely on patient interviews. But interviews and other similar measures, such as compliance ratings by physicians or therapy outcomes, may be inaccurate or biased.[16] However, they are more accurate than suspected.[12]

A patient's compliance pattern may change over time. Fluctuations in medication concentration during times of constant prescribed dose—beyond those expected from assay error or pharmacologic fluctuations—may reflect noncompliance with the prescribed regimen. The degree of fluctuation can be cal-

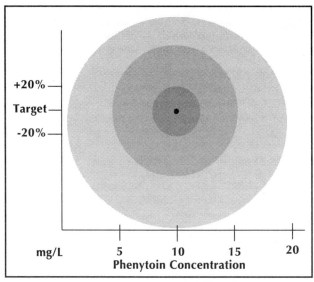

Figure 3—Representation of allowable variability over time if the target level of phenytoin is 10 mg/L. Levels between 8 and 12 mg/L are within the 20% fluctuation observed in compliant patients. Levels below 5.5 mg/L and above 14.5 mg/L are usually associated with noncompliance.

culated using the coefficient of variation (CV), as described in the equation in Figure 2.

A number of studies have evaluated variability of serial phenytoin and carbamazepine concentrations in various settings. In a study of phenytoin, patients in a residential facility were found to have CV values of less than 10%.[17] In compliant patients in an outpatient study of bioavailability, where samples were obtained every 2 weeks and compliance was monitored by pill counts and interviews, the CV of phenytoin was less than 20%.[17] A few of these patients reported missing an occasional dose several days before the blood sample was taken. This did not significantly affect the CV. In this same study, sequential epilepsy clinic patients were asked about compliance; there was a strong correlation between reported noncompliance and a high CV. Data from rigorous studies indi-

Table 4:   Examples of Patients From the MINCEP Clinic
Illustrating Use of Variability in Serial Levels
to Determine Compliance

Pt#	Dates of Visits	Medication	Daily Dose	Level mg/L	
251	9-28-88	PHT	460 mg	20.8	Mean=23.1
	7-12-89	PHT	460 mg	25.1	± 20%=4.6
	1-10-90	PHT	460 mg	23.3	Compliant
	10-24-90	PHT	460 mg	13.1*	range=
					18.5 to 27.7
80	2-28-89	CBZ	2000 mg	7.2	Mean=8.6
	5-2-89	CBZ	2000 mg	9.0	± 20%=1.8
	10-31-89	CBZ	2000 mg	9.6	Compliant
	2-12-91	CBZ	2000 mg	5.0*	range=
					6.5 to 10.4

* Out of range, probable noncompliance
PHT=phenytoin
CBZ=carbamazepine

cate that most compliant patients had CV below 20%[18] for carbamazepine.

Based on this experience, we have adopted the guideline of the percent deviation from the mean of two or more levels to aid in evaluation of noncompliance. Although calculation of the CV is more accurate, a determination of the percent deviation is simpler and more practical for clinical use. In general, deviation of 20% or less from the mean of previous phenytoin, carbamazepine, or valproate concentrations is evidence for adequate compliant behavior. A patient can attain the 20% limit even if he or she misses an occasional dose (Figure 3). Values between 20% to 45% should raise strong suspicions of noncompliance. Values deviating more than 45% are almost always associated with noncompliance. The larger the percentage, the more marked the noncompliance—assuming the absence of any factors altering the pharmacokinetics, such as new medication, illness, or altered bioavailability.

Generally, blood samples should be drawn at the same time relative to the dose to be useful for compliance measurements. In a clinic setting, this can be accomplished by always scheduling appointments for the same time of day. Our limit is plus

Table 5: Strategies to Improve Patient Compliance

Education

- Explain diagnosis and treatment plan
- Discuss the timetable for follow-up
- Provide pamphlets or video presentations
- Arrange for staff to help patient and family understand
- Explain how to implement treatment

Dosing

- Reduce the number of medications
- Reduce the number of doses taken each day
- Provide a dose checklist
- Provide a pill box with a daily compartment or alarm reminder

Clinic Visits

- Increase the frequency of visits
- Designate a specific clinic staff person for contacts

---

or minus 1 hour. This can be attained most of the time. For example, a person with a 3 PM examination usually has blood drawn by 3:30 PM, but any time between 2:30 PM and 4:30 PM is acceptable.

Serial measurements of AED levels are a powerful tool for detecting noncompliance (Table 4). With increasing legal pressure on physicians to certify driving licenses or workplace safety for patients with epilepsy, knowing that a patient is compliant becomes critical. Thus, even if a patient's AED concentrations fall within the usual therapeutic range, but vary from the high to the low end, noncompliant behavior must be suspected. That patient may be at increased risk for intermittent toxicity or seizures.

Measurement of serial blood levels is relatively crude compared with the use of a device that records each opening of a medication container daily. Such a device can detect noncompliant behavior lasting only a few days between clinic visits or blood level measurements.[10] However, use of this method is limited now to clinical research because of its cost.

Psychosocial Aspects of Compliance

Another aspect of compliance is intention, which can be patient controlled or structural. Patient noncompliance can be rational or irrational. Rational noncompliance usually arises from a well-defined, logical, and consistent belief system—eg, the pregnant woman who decides to suspend use of AEDs because of concerns about teratogenicity. Although the accuracy of the risk/benefit calculation might be open to question, the decision is founded in logic.

An example of an irrational belief system is one in which a patient believes that seizures are influenced by the moon, and therefore that medications are not needed during certain lunar phases.

Structural reasons for noncompliance are outside a patient's control. For example, a patient who developed epilepsy after trauma to the temporal lobes would have memory dysfunction, leading to difficulty in remembering a medication schedule.

Strategies to Improve Compliance

Some life-style habits can precipitate seizures, such as irregular sleep patterns, alcohol or drug abuse, exposure to psychological stress, or, for photosensitive individuals, exposure to light. Patients may be compliant with a medication regimen but still experience excessive seizures because they are exposed to these risk factors.

Some strategies for improving compliance are reviewed by Shope[9] and are listed in Table 5. The most important factor is correctly identifying the underlying cause of noncompliance. Each patient must be considered individually. If the intention toward compliance is being thwarted by external factors, these must be addressed. For example, a patient whose limited financial resources preclude the purchase of expensive medications might be switched to a less costly drug. In contrast, education may be the key if a patient does not understand the short half-lives of AEDs and has not been informed about the importance of taking medication regularly.

References

1. Kupferberg HF: Quantitative estimates of diphenylhydantoin, primidone, and phenobarbital in plasma by gas-liquid chromatography. *Clin Chim Acta* 1970;29:282-288.

2. Wad N: Simultaneous determination of 11 antiepileptic compounds in serum by high-performance liquid chromatography. *J Chromatogr* 1984;305:127-133.

3. Graves NM, Holmes GB, Leppik IE, et al: Quantitative determination of phenytoin and phenobarbital in capillary blood by Ames Seralyzer. *Epilepsia* 1987;28:713-716.

4. Leppik IE, Oles KS, Sheehan ML, et al: Phenytoin and phenobarbital concentrations in serum: a comparison of Ames Seralyzer with GLC, TDX, and EMIT. *Ther Drug Monit* 1989;1:73-78.

5. Tyrer JH, Eadie MJ, Sutherland JM, et al: Outbreak of anticonvulsant intoxication in an Australian city. *Br Med J* 1970;4:271-273.

6. Rosenbaum DH, Rowan AJ, Tuchman L, et al: Comparative bioavailability of a generic phenytoin and Dilantin. *Epilepsia* 1994;35(3):656-660.

7. Dosing M: Effect of acute and chronic exercise on hepatic drug metabolism. *Clin Pharmacokinet* 1985;10:426-431.

8. Levy RH, Unadkat JD: General principles: drug absorption, distribution and elimination. In: Levy RH, Dreifuss FE, Mattson RH, et al, eds. *Antiepileptic Drugs.* 3rd ed. New York, NY, Raven Press, 1989, pp 1-22.

9. Leppik IE, Schmidt D, eds: Summary of the First International Workshop on Compliance in Epilepsy. *Epilepsy Res* 1988;1(suppl):179-182.

10. Shope J: Intervention to improve compliance with pediatric anticonvulsant therapy. *Patient Couns Health Educ* 1980;21:135-141.

11. Cramer JA, Mattson RH, Prevey ML, et al: How often is medication taken as prescribed? A novel assessment technique. *JAMA* 1989;261:3273-3277.

12. Green LW, Simons-Morton D: Denial, delay, and disappointment: discovering and overcoming the causes of drug errors and missed appointments. *Epilepsy Res* 1988;1(suppl):7-22.

13. Cranford RE, Leppik IE, Patrick B: Intravenous phenytoin: clinical and pharmacokinetic aspects. *Neurology* 1978;28:874-880.

14. Stanaway L, Lambie DG, Johnson RH: Noncompliance with anticonvulsant therapy as a cause for seizures. *N Z Med J* 1985;98:150-152.

15. Leppik IE, Ramani V, Sawchuk RJ, et al: Increased clearance of phenytoin during infectious mononucleosis. *N Engl J Med* 1979;300:481-482.

16. Mushlin AI, Appel FA: Diagnosing potential noncompliance. Physicians' ability in a behavioral dimension of medical care. *Arch Intern Med* 1977;137:318-321.

17. Leppik IE, Cloyd JC, Sawchuk RJ, et al: Compliance and variability of plasma phenytoin levels in epileptic patients. *Ther Drug Monit* 1979;1:475-483.

18. Graves NM, Holmes GB, Leppik IE: Compliant populations: variability in serum concentrations. *Epilepsy Res* 1988;1(suppl):91-99.

Chapter 9

Serious Adverse Reactions and Laboratory Testing

As the public becomes increasingly concerned about the cost of health care, physicians can expect to feel more pressure to cut costs. While facing these pressures, physicians must also consider the overall cost to the patient and to society of not performing necessary laboratory testing. However, the need and cost-effectiveness for routine laboratory testing to detect serious adverse effects to all antiepileptic drugs has come under question.[1,2]

Serious reactions to antiseizure medications are uncommon. They include hepatotoxicity, bone marrow suppression, pancreatitis, exfoliative dermatitis, and others, which, if not detected in time, may be fatal. Because of the perceived medicolegal climate, much emphasis has been placed on routine monitoring of hepatic and hematopoietic factors. On the other hand, Canadian medical societies have discouraged the use of routine testing.[1]

The popularity of laboratory monitoring is based on the assumption that subclinical hepatitis or hematopoietic dysfunction can be detected. But elevations of hepatic enzymes of twice the "normal" range are not unusual, and mild leukopenia is a common side effect in patients treated with antiepileptic drugs (AEDs). In addition to being costly, laboratory testing may be misleading, provoke further testing, or lead to inappropriate discontinuation of medication.

The cost of performing routine laboratory testing is considerable. If one assumes that 2.8 million persons are being treated for epilepsy in the United States, that a set of hematologic and hepatic tests costs $50, and that the test is repeated three times a year for each patient, the cumulative cost would be $420 million. This greatly exceeds the total annual funds being spent on research for epilepsy.

There are two reasons for the great reluctance in the United States to abandon routine laboratory monitoring. First, there is the misperception that such testing is useful in detecting a serious adverse event early enough to prevent a fatal outcome. Second, there is the real concern that the medicolegal consequences of not following community practice standards could be very severe. However, support is growing in the literature for abandonment of routine monitoring and for more specific risk-assessment evaluations.[1,3]

Rate of Adverse Effects

The precise frequency of serious drug effects from antiseizure medications is difficult to determine because of inadequate postmarketing surveillance. Most of the information available comes from two sources: reports in the medical literature and information from drug manufacturers supplied to the United States Food and Drug Administration.

Tables 1 and 2 list the approximate number of cases of life-threatening reactions attributable to specific antiepileptic medications in the United States, derived from the medical literature. Although crude, this number underscores the infrequent occurrence of serious reactions. Felbamate is the one exception; its rate for aplastic anemia is approximately 1 in 5,000 and for hepatitis is approximately 1 in 10,000.

Carbamazepine was considered to be associated with a high risk of aplastic anemia but in a thorough review using estimated number of persons exposed per year,[4] a rate of 2 cases of aplastic anemia for 575,000 treated persons and 1 fatality was calculated. Aplastic anemia has rarely been reported in association with valproate, and well-documented cases of aplastic anemia in phenobarbital or other antiepileptic medications are rare.

A pattern emerges for hepatitis. The highest risk group is infants exposed to valproate in the context of polypharmacy.[5] This may result from the fact that valproate metabolism depends on both cytoplasmic and mitochondrial systems, and the relative production of hepatotoxic metabolites is influenced by the amount of drug passing through each system. The proportion of cytoplasmic and mitochondrial metabolism may be influenced by comedication and changes with age. In addition, the existence of metabolic or neurologic disorders poses a significant risk.[6] The actual number of fatal hepatitis cases attributable to phenytoin is difficult to determine, but the overall number may be approximately 50. Carbamazepine and other medications appear to have a lower

Table 1: Serious Idiosyncratic Reactions to Antiepileptic Medications, Listed in Order of Concern

Reaction	AED	Approximate Rate
Aplastic anemia	felbamate	1/5,000
	carbamazepine	2/575,000
	phenytoin	A
	barbiturates	A
Hepatitis	felbamate	1/10,000
	valproate	see Table 2
	phenytoin	A
	carbamazepine	A
	barbiturates	A
Pancreatitis	valproate	A
Serious rashes	lamotrigine	1/100 (in children) 3/1,000 (in adults)
	phenytoin	A
	carbamazepine	A
	valproate	A
Renal calculi	topiramate	1/100
	zonisamide	1/100

A= higher than spontaneous occurrence, but probably less than 1/500,000

Table 2: Approximate Rate of Occurrence of Fatal Hepatitis from Valproate

Age	Monotherapy	Polytherapy
infant	1/7,000	1/500
child	1/9,000	1/6,500
adult	0	1/22,000

* Data from Dreifuss et al.[5]

rate of occurrence of hepatitis. Thus, the only group at major risk are infants on valproate[7]; adults receiving valproate or other antiseizure medications are at very low risk.

Other potentially fatal adverse reactions include pancreatitis, serum sickness reaction, Stevens-Johnson syndrome, and other rare complications. Routine laboratory testing for pan-

Table 3:	Laboratory Parameters: Normal Ranges and Threshold ("Panic") Values for Antiseizure Medications	
Hematologic	**Normal Range**	**"Panic" Values**
WBC, total	4,500–10,000/mm^3	below 2.0 mm^3
Neutrophils	1,500–6,700/mm^3	below 1.0 mm^3
Eosinophils	200–500/mm^3	above 600/mm^3 (or 10% or more of WBC)
Platelets	150,000–350,000/mm^3	below 50 mm^3
RBC	3.8 million–5 million/mm^3	below 3200 mm^3
Hemoglobin	11.5–15.0 g/dL	below 10.0 g/dL
Hematocrit	34%–44%	below 28%
Mean RBC volume	83–94 μm^3	above 100 μm^3
Mean RBC Hb	28–32 pg	above 35 pg
Hepatic		
Transaminase (SGOT)	15–40 units/L	above 100 units/L
Transaminase (SGPT)	9–31 units/L	above 100 units/L
LDH	60–200 units/L	above 600 units/L
Alk phosphatase	30–115 units/L	above 300 units/L
γ-glutamyltransferase (GGT)	0–65 units/L	above 800 units/L
Bilirubin, total	0.2–1.2 mg/dL	above 1.5 mg/dL
Other		
Sodium	135–145 mEq/L	below 128 mEq/L
Amylase	may vary	3 x laboratory normal

creatitis is unnecessary because clinical symptoms of abdominal pain, anorexia, etc, are dramatic and will lead to specific confirmatory tests. For the others, clinical skills are more diagnostic than laboratory findings.

Problem of False Positives

Table 3 is a list of laboratory tests performed routinely. The "panic" values are those that trigger an immediate re-

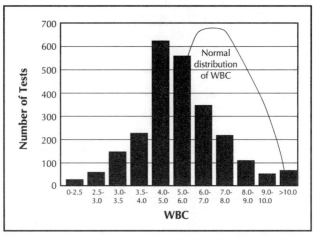

Figure 1—Histogram of approximately 2,500 WBC values from patients with epilepsy followed at MINCEP over 2 years. Laboratory normal values are from 4.5 to 10.0.

sponse from the laboratory, and may be grounds for considering discontinuation of the drug.

Use of antiseizure medications often leads to values outside of the laboratory normal ranges. A study of 610 persons with epilepsy between 20 and 40 years of age evaluated the effect of long-term treatment on various laboratory parameters.[8] The findings were that leukocyte counts were significantly lower, with a specific lowering of lymphocytes. Also, persistent macrocytosis without anemia was noted. In a review of approximately 2,500 white blood cell (WBC) counts in the MINCEP population of more than 1,100 patients with epilepsy receiving primarily valproate, phenytoin, and/or carbamazepine, more than 17% had WBC counts below 4,000/cm^3, and eight had a WBC count below 2,500 (1,800 to 2,400)/cm^3.[9] These eight were clinically asymptomatic and, in two cases, the physician discontinued carbamazepine based on laboratory findings. In one patient with AIDS and epilepsy, zidovudine (AZT) was discontinued and the WBC count normalized. In five cases, no change occurred in treatment. The lowest WBC count was 1,800 cm^3. The population with epilepsy had a lower WBC count histogram, but this lowering

Table 4: Package Insert Recommendations for Monitoring Laboratory Parameters When Using AEDs

Carbamazepine (Novartis)	"Complete pretreatment blood counts, including platelets and possibly reticulocytes and serum iron, should be obtained as a baseline. If a patient in the course of treatment exhibits low or decreased white blood cell or platelet counts, the patient should be monitored closely. Baseline and periodic evaluations of liver function, particularly in patients with a history of liver disease, must be performed during treatment with this drug."
Felbamate (Wallace)	"Full hematologic evaluations should be performed before Felbatol® therapy, frequently during therapy, and for a significant period of time after discontinuation of therapy. While it might appear prudent to perform frequent CBCs in patients continuing on this drug, there is no evidence that such monitoring will allow early detection of marrow suppression before aplastic anemia occurs. Complete pretreatment blood counts, including platelets and reticulocytes, should be obtained as a baseline. If any hematologic abnormalities are detected during the course of treatment, immediate consultation with a hematologist is advised. Liver function testing (ALT, AST, bilirubin) should be done before Felbatol® is started and at 1- to 2- week intervals while the patient is taking Felbatol®."
Gabapentin (Parke-Davis)	"Clinical trials do not indicate that routine monitoring of clinical laboratory parameters is necessary."
Lamotrigine (Glaxo Wellcome)	No specific recommendations
Levetiracetam (UCB Pharma)	No specific recommendations

(continued on next page)

Table 4: Package Insert Recommendations for Monitoring Laboratory Parameters When Using AEDs *(continued)*

Oxcarbazepine (Novartis)	No specific recommendations
Phenytoin (Parke-Davis)	No specific recommendations
Tiagabine (Abbott)	No specific recommendations
Topiramate (Ortho-McNeil)	No specific recommendations
Valproate (Abbott)	"Liver function tests should be performed prior to therapy and at frequent intervals thereafter, especially during the first 6 months. However, physicians should not rely totally on serum biochemistry since these tests may not be abnormal in all instances..."
Zonisamide (Elan)	No specific recommendations

did not appear to be associated with any clinical problems (Figure 1). Other reports have documented transient leukopenia in up to 12% of adults and children treated with carbamazepine.[10]

γ-Glutamyltransferase (GGT) levels are markedly elevated in patients with epilepsy[8] and do not signal hepatic dysfunction. Serum glutamic oxaloacetic transaminase (SGOT, same as aspartate transaminase [AST]) levels may be more reliable. In the MINCEP database,[9] approximately 33% of values from more than 1,100 patients were above normal; 12 had SGOT (AST) values above 100 IU (normal = 10 to 35). In eight cases, the elevations were sporadic, that is, the values were in the usual range when the test was repeated. In four cases, all on valproate, the medication dose was decreased, and in one it was discontinued. All four had clinical symptoms of loss of appetite, malaise, or nausea, which had alerted the clinician to possible problems that led to testing.

> **Table 5: Tests to Be Done Before Treatment With Antiseizure Medications**
>
> - CBC, differential, platelets
> - Serum chemistry to include liver enzymes, protein, creatinine, electrolytes
> - For topiramate and zonisamide, urine analysis with microscopic examination

Thus, from the MINCEP database of more than 5,000 visits, involving more than 1,100 patients who were followed for 24 months, the incidence of WBC counts of less than $2,500/cm^3$ was 6.6 per 1,000 patients.[9] The rate for "panic" SGOT elevations was higher. Nevertheless, clinical symptoms led to tests that uncovered abnormal values. Thus, overall, routine testing alone uncovered only two asymptomatic "panic" values that led to modification of therapy. The approximate total cost of these tests was $125,000. Based on these figures, it is reasonable to conclude that the cost effectiveness of routine laboratory testing is very questionable. Most "panic" values were false-positives in the sense that they did not lead to modification of treatment, but only to additional testing.

Camfield et al[3] reported similar results from a smaller series. They performed serial testing at initiation of treatment, at 1, 3, and 6 months, and then every 6 months. There were no serious clinical reactions, but laboratory testing was repeated in 6% of patients to confirm abnormal but clinically insignificant results. In a study of 662 adults in whom treatment was initiated with phenytoin, carbamazepine, phenobarbital, or primidone, no clinically significant abnormalities were detected after 6 months.[11]

Alternatives to Routine Blood Monitoring

Table 4 lists the current recommendations in the product package inserts for monitoring laboratory results of antiepileptic drugs. The present recommendations are less strict than found in previous editions. With the exception of felbamate, none of the other drugs need to be monitored frequently.[12] Screening laboratory testing should be performed to detect any underlying problems before initiating therapy with antiseizure medications. These tests could uncover spe-

135

cific problems that, if they develop further, may be incorrectly attributed to the medication (Table 5).

Patients in a high-risk group and those unable to communicate must be monitored more closely. The most efficient monitoring system is a high degree of awareness of symptoms that portend serious complications, patient awareness of these, and rapid assessment of any problems that suggest a rare but potentially fatal complication.

References

1. Pellock JM, Willmore LJ: A rational guide to routine blood monitoring in patients receiving antiepileptic drugs. *Neurology* 1991;41:961-964.

2. Wyllie E, Wyllie R: Routine laboratory monitoring for serious adverse effects of antiepileptic medications: the controversy. *Epilepsia* 1991;32(suppl 5):S74-S79.

3. Camfield P, Camfield C, Dooley J, et al: Routine screening of blood and urine for severe reactions to anticonvulsant drugs in asymptomatic patients is of doubtful value. *Can Med Assoc J* 1989;140:1303-1305.

4. Seetharam MN, Pellock JM: Risk-benefit assessment of carbamazepine in children. *Drug Saf* 1991;6:148-158.

5. Dreifuss FE, Langer DH, Moline KA, et al: Valproic acid hepatic fatalities. II. U.S. experience since 1984. *Neurology* 1989;39:201-207.

6. Willmore LJ, Triggs WJ, Pellock JM: Valproate toxicity: risk-screening strategies. *Child Neurol* 1991;6:3-6.

7. Scheffner D, Konig S, Rauterberg-Ruland I, et al: Fatal liver failure in 16 children with valproate therapy. *Epilepsia* 1988;29:530-542.

8. Krause KH: Side effects of antiepileptic drugs in long-term treatment. *Klin Wochenschr* 1988;66:601-604.

9. Leppik IE, Jacobs MP, Loewenson RB, et al: Detection of adverse events by routine laboratory testing. *Epilepsia* 1990;31(5):640.

10. Pellock JM: Carbamazepine side effects in children and adults. *Epilepsia* 1987;28(suppl 3):S64-S70.

11. Mattson RH, Cramer JA, Collins JF, et al: Connective tissue changes, hypersensitivity rash and blood laboratory test changes associated with antiepileptic drug therapy. *Ann Neurol* 1986;20:119-120.

12. Leppik IE, Wolff DL: The place of felbamate in the treatment of epilepsy. *CNS Drugs* 1995;4:294-301.

Chapter 10

Pregnancy and Epilepsy

A pproximately 20,000 births occur among women with epilepsy each year in the United States. Caring for women with epilepsy who are pregnant or contemplating pregnancy raises a number of issues about proper treatment. These include the effect of pregnancy on seizure frequency, the effect of seizures on the fetus, the effect of antiepileptic drugs on the growth and development of the fetus, problems with labor and delivery, the implications for breast-feeding, and the ability of a mother with seizures to care for her child.

The most important aspect in caring for a woman with epilepsy is discussing issues before pregnancy. Decisions regarding treatment should consider that conception may occur before the next patient/physician interaction. Although there is a perception that women with epilepsy are at very high risk for adverse outcomes of pregnancy, this presumption is not supported by large studies.[1,2]

Seizure Frequency During Pregnancy

In one study of 153 pregnancies in 59 women with epilepsy, seizures increased during 45% of pregnancies, decreased during 5%, and showed no change during 50%.[3] In a review of the literature describing 2,165 pregnancies, 24% were found to experience an increase in seizures, 23% a decrease, and 53% no change.[4] That same study found 12 cases of status epilepticus, the most frightening and potentially serious exacerbation of seizures during pregnancy.[4] In another review of pregnant women with epilepsy, 29 cases of status epilepticus were identified. Nine women died, as did 14 of the fetuses.[5]

Pregnancy is associated with a number of physiologic, endocrinologic, and psychological changes, any or all of which might contribute to lowering the seizure threshold. Women often gain weight during pregnancy, some of which may be caused by increased retention of water and sodium. Some have postulated that these might be responsible for the increase in seizure frequency. However, studies in women with exacerbation of seizures during their menstrual cycles (catamenial epilepsy) have not shown a correlation between seizure frequency, body weight, and total body water.

Plasma progesterone and estradiol levels gradually increase during pregnancy. Chorionic gonadotropin peaks in the first trimester and then drops during the end of the pregnancy. A number of animal models of epilepsy have demonstrated that estrogen has the ability to increase animals' susceptibility to maximal electroshock seizures. Furthermore, focal spikes increase and clinical seizures are exacerbated by intravenous injection of estrogen. However, progesterone may decrease seizure susceptibility in experimental animals and in patients. No comprehensive studies have been done correlating women's endocrinologic changes during pregnancy with alteration in seizure frequency.

The best predictor of seizure frequency during pregnancy appears to be seizure frequency before pregnancy. Almost all patients who had more than one seizure per month in one study had an increase in seizures during pregnancy, whereas women having less than one seizure every 9 months did not experience an increase during pregnancy.[3] Psychological stress factors, such as anxiety leading to lack of sleep, have been postulated as important in lowering seizure threshold.

The major factor may be poor compliance in taking antiepileptic medication. In a group of 125 Japanese women, 27% considered to be poorly compliant had a significant increase in seizure frequency during pregnancy.[6] In a study of 136 German women, noncompliance with medication was considered to be the major factor in aggravating seizure frequency during pregnancy.[7]

Risks to the Offspring

The developing fetus in an epileptic patient is exposed to two sources of risk: the metabolic and mechanical stresses from the generalized tonic-clonic seizures, and the problems caused by antiepileptic medications and their metabolites. Lowering risks of teratogenicity by reducing medication may lead to a greater risk for seizures, which can also harm the fetus. Abrupt discontinuation may precipitate seizures or status epilepticus. Balancing risk from medications against risk from increased seizures requires the exercise of careful judgment based on the most current information.

Effect of Seizures on the Fetus

Intracranial hemorrhage in utero following a maternal seizure can occur. In one well-documented case, a 28-year-old woman had a generalized seizure during the 19th week of gestation. A second seizure occurred in the 28th week of gestation after she missed several doses of medication. After the third seizure, between the 32nd and 33rd week of gestation, the patient felt decreased fetal movement. A sonogram revealed intracerebral hemorrhage with moderate hydrocephalus. There was no evidence of fetal cardiac activity or body motion. Eight days after the second seizure, labor was induced and the patient delivered a stillborn, macerated male weighing 1,815 g.[8]

Another dramatic report describes a woman who was being monitored during spontaneous labor at term. A spiral electrode had been attached to the fetal scalp for recording the fetal heart rate. Forty-three minutes before delivery, when her cervix was dilated to 6 cm, the patient unexpectedly had a generalized tonic-clonic seizure, lasting 2.5 minutes. Immediately after the seizure, the patient became cyanotic and received 10 mg of diazepam intravenously. Fetal heart rate decelerated to less than 120 beats per minute for more than 13 minutes after the seizure. Twenty-nine minutes after the generalized seizure, late deceleration bradycardia was still observed, and therefore, a cesarean section was performed. Total phenytoin concentration in maternal venous blood was only 0.9 mg/L, suggesting patient noncompliance.[9] Another monitored birth recorded a fetal heart beat of less than 100 after a brief seizure.

These observations indicate that a human fetus clearly becomes asphyctic, as judged by the fetal heart monitoring during and after generalized tonic-clonic seizures. Deceleration in heart rate can persist for some time and has the potential of damaging the infant's development.

While case reports are dramatic, population-based studies give a picture of the extent of the problem. The Collaborative Perinatal Project of the National Institutes of Health found that 4.4 women per 1,000 of approximately 45,000 women had one or more seizures during pregnancy.[10] The rate of stillbirths in women with seizures (not including eclampsia) was 5.14%, significantly higher than the 2.4% in women with epi-

Table 1:   Outcomes of Pregnancy From Two Large Population-Based Studies

	Births	Malformations	Relative Risk	
Australian Study [1]				
Mothers with diabetes	225	19	(8.4%)*	2.5
Mothers with epilepsy	244	9	(3.7%)	1.1
All other mothers	62,265	2,009	(3.4%)	1.0
Norwegian Study [2]				
Mothers with epilepsy	3,879	170	(4.4%)*	1.25
Control births	3,879	136	(3.5%)	1.0

* statistically significant difference

[1] Used with permission, Stanley FJ, et al.

[2] Used with permission, Bjerkedal T: *Epilepsy, Pregnancy, and the Child.* New York, Raven Press, 1982, pp 289-295.

lepsy but no seizures during the pregnancy. Head circumference two standard deviations or more below the mean was significantly greater in women who had a seizure during pregnancy, as was the rate for mixed cerebral palsy and for mental retardation. Thus, it is evident from this large study that seizures occurring during pregnancy can impair fetal development and cause stillbirth.

Complex partial seizures may result in accidents or injuries that may harm the mother, and thus indirectly harm the fetus. An example would be major burns suffered by a pregnant woman as a consequence of a complex partial seizure that required prolonged treatment with a number of drugs. Such a case would subject the fetus to all of the physiologic changes that occur with extensive third-degree burns and to the risks from the multiple drugs used to treat them. Thus, the goal of therapy should be to achieve control of all seizures during pregnancy.

Fetal Maldevelopment

The risks of malformations in the offspring of women with epilepsy have been a topic of much debate in the literature.

Generally, smaller, older, less well-controlled studies have shown higher rates than larger, population-based, case-controlled studies.

One study that was limited to evaluating congenital heart defects found that of 2,461 live children born to people with epilepsy, the rate of malformation was similar in mothers with epilepsy, in fathers with epilepsy, and in the control population. Thus, the authors concluded that antiepileptic treatment is not a major etiologic factor in congenital heart defects in the offspring of parents with epilepsy.[12] Two larger population-based studies have shown no significant risk, while another found a small but statistically significant risk[1,2] (Table 1).

The teratogenic potential of phenytoin has been the subject of much debate. One early study reported a malformation rate of 27.3%. A large, well-controlled study comparing 1,411 children born to mothers with epilepsy using antiepileptic drugs during the first trimester to 2,000 matched controls has shed considerable light on the issue of malformations.[13] The study population was large enough to permit statistically meaningful comparisons between the major antiepileptic drugs. The most interesting finding was that in contrast to earlier, smaller studies, phenytoin monotherapy was not associated with an increased risk for major malformations (Table 2).

Of 151 children born to mothers being treated with phenytoin, only one had a major malformation (cleft lip, hypospadias, and sacral defect).[13] This finding led the authors to conclude that "phenytoin monotherapy might be less teratogenic than thought before."[13] This finding is also supported by a prospective controlled study that found distal digital hypoplasia as the only minor malformation that could be linked to phenytoin.[14]

A syndrome once thought to be specific to phenytoin has been called the fetal hydantoin syndrome.[15] Its features are similar to the fetal alcohol syndrome and consist of major and minor congenital anomalies. The major anomalies include microcephaly, growth retardation, and impaired intellectual functioning. Minor anomalies include strabismus, ptosis, ocular hypertelorism, broad and/or distal phalanges with or without nail hypoplasia, hyperextensible joints, hypotonia, pilonidal sinus, inguinal hernia, umbilical hernia, abnormal dermatoglyphic patterns, and minor club deformities of the feet. These may lead to a characteristic facial appearance. Many of the features seen in the fetal hydantoin syndrome may also be seen with the use of barbiturates.[16] These features have also been observed with all other antiepileptic drugs. The term *fetal antiepileptic drug syndrome* is more appropriate. However, this 'syndrome' has been reported only in isolated case reports, and has not been found in the larger, controlled studies,[13,14] raising doubt about its specificity to antiepileptic drugs.

Significant neural tube defects associated with valproate have been reported. Data from a registry of spina bifida and anencephaly revealed that these defects occurred in a much higher frequency than expected in children of mothers being treated with valproate.[17] In one study of 12 children born to 11 epileptic mothers, two children were born with microcephaly.[18] Thus, valproate may have a specific teratogenic effect. In a large, controlled study, 9 out of 159 children born to mothers receiving valproate as monotherapy had major malformations, mostly spina bifida (Table 2). This effect was dose related and was most common with the highest doses.[13]

Carbamazepine also poses a risk for spina bifida. One recent study concluded that carbamazepine has a 0.5% to 1% risk for this malformation. A large, controlled study found carbamazepine to be the second most teratogenic of the common antiepileptic drugs (Table 2).[13,19]

Primidone appears to be more teratogenic than phenobarbital by itself.[20] But claims that barbiturates are less teratogenic than other antiepileptic drugs, with the exception of trimethadione, cannot be substantiated by available literature.

Most studies show that the risk of malformations increases with the number of drugs used (Table 2).[13,21] However, seizures may also play a role. For example, in one study, the incidence of malformation was the highest (12.7%) in medicated patients who had seizures during pregnancy.[21] Thus, the highest risk of fetal injury occurs in women whose seizures are incompletely controlled even with multiple drug use.

There appears to be a strong association between maternal folic acid insufficiency and fetal malformations, spontaneous abortion, and placental abruption. A retrospective study

Table 2:	Antiepileptic Drugs and Major Malformations Observed in a Large Study of 2,000 Controls and 1,411 Children Born to Mothers With Epilepsy Using Antiepileptic Drugs[13]		
Group	**N**	**%**	**Risk Ratio**
Control	29/2,000	1	1.0
Monotherapy			
phenytoin	1/151	1	0.5
carbamazepine	14/376	4	2.6*
valproate	9/159	6	4.1*
Polytherapy			
phenytoin	6/209	3	2.0
benzodiazepines	6/106	6	4.1*
carbamazepine	12/225	5	3.8*
valproate	8/136	5	3.7*
caffeine	5/75	7	4.9*
any 2 drugs	16/342	5	3.3*
any 3 drugs	4/91	4	3.1*
any 4 drugs	4/52	8	5.9*

*Statistically significantly different from control

examining the effect of folic acid supplementation on congenital malformations from antiepileptic drugs reported that 66 children born to women who received antiepileptic drugs without folic acid had a 15% rate of malformation. These consisted of heart disease, cleft lip and palate, neural tube defects, and skeletal abnormalities. A prospective study by the same investigators found that 33 infants born to 22 epileptic women taking folic acid supplements were without congenital malformations and were of normal body weight. Based on these dramatic results, a recommendation for folic acid supplementation during pregnancy was made.[22] A study by Dansky[11] supports these results. Use of folic acid supplement during pregnancy is recommended (from 0.8 to 5 mg/day).

A confounding variable is the genetic influence on malformations. One study indicated that children born to fathers with epilepsy had a higher rate of malformations than did controls, but other studies are needed to confirm these findings.

It appears, then, that although some studies have reported exceedingly high rates of malformations in women with epilepsy, the weight of the evidence, especially from larger, well-controlled studies, is that the offspring of women with epilepsy have a 1% to 2% risk above baseline of malformations. While some of the increased risk is attributable to antiepileptic drugs, the more likely cause is the complex interaction of genetic factors and environmental factors (drugs, vitamin deficiencies, etc) working in concert. Little data are available regarding human teratogenicity of the newer AEDs. However, animal studies in equivalent species have shown that gabapentin, lamotrigine, levetiracetam, and felbamate do not have significant teratogenicity.

A guideline adopted by the American Epilepsy Society and the Academy of Neurology states that the AEDs most effective for treatment of the specific epilepsy syndrome be used.

Antiepileptic Drug Pharmacokinetics

Drug absorption. Gastric tone and motility are reduced during pregnancy, resulting in delayed emptying of the stomach. Antacids are frequently prescribed during pregnancy. Dimethicone, a common constituent of antacids, reduces phenytoin absorption by 71%, and kaolin reduces it by 60%, whereas magnesium trisilicate has a negligible effect.[23] Nausea and vomiting are other symptoms during pregnancy that affect drug ingestion and absorption, especially during the first trimester.

Metabolism. Pregnancy prompts changes in almost every aspect of metabolism. A number of changes occur in the liver during pregnancy, and these may affect drug metabolism. The rising concentrations of steroids increase the capacity for hydroxylation, and these substances are competitive inhibitors of microsomal oxidases for drugs such as ethylmorphine or hexobarbitone, and may reduce their elimination.

The fetoplacental unit increases the volume of distribution of drugs that is administered to the mother and also contributes to drug metabolism. However, such fetal metabolism usually has no clinically discernible effect on maternal drug concentrations because the fetal circulation is so small compared to the maternal circulation.

Protein Binding. Some antiepileptic medications are highly protein bound. Many studies conducted in vitro have shown that pregnancy significantly decreases the plasma protein binding of phenytoin, phenobarbital, valproate, and diazepam.

Specific Antiepileptic Drugs

Phenytoin concentrations may decrease significantly during pregnancy. Half-lives of phenytoin during pregnancy have been reported to be decreased by as much as 50%. In a prospective study, plasma phenytoin levels were measured during the course of pregnancy in 100 women. Doses were increased when levels fell, and the dose related to level was used to calculate the apparent clearance. Phenytoin clearance increased gradually during the first 32 weeks of pregnancy, reached twice the preconception value during the last 8 weeks, and began to return to normal during the 12-week period after pregnancy.[24]

Phenytoin is a weak acid and is poorly soluble in water. Its pK_a is in the range of 8.3 to 9.2. It is not absorbed in the stomach, but is absorbed in the upper small intestine, and to a lesser degree in the lower small intestine. Very little is absorbed in the cecum or large intestine. Malabsorption may also be related to the use of antacids, which can decrease the amount of phenytoin in solution by forming insoluble complexes.

Phenytoin is avidly bound by plasma protein. Protein binding is greatly influenced by pregnancy in both humans and experimental animals.[25] In normal women 8 to 15 weeks pregnant, phenytoin binding measured in vitro is within normal limits. However, women progressing beyond the 16th week of gestation have decreased binding of phenytoin to plasma proteins. This change in binding persists for at least 5 days after delivery and returns to normal 5 to 7 weeks postpartum.[26]

These in vitro experiments have been verified by studies of women receiving phenytoin who were followed through pregnancy. This change in protein binding explains in part the observed decrease in total phenytoin concentrations during pregnancy. One study of six women with epilepsy found that the total serum phenytoin concentration was considerably lower the day of delivery. Most of this decrease was explained by a drop in plasma protein binding, but there was a decrease in the unbound concentration, indicating that both increased clearance and binding displacement were responsible. The unbound fraction of phenytoin in pregnant women correlates negatively with serum albumin concentrations[26] and positively with gestational age. Studies of unbound drug concentrations in maternal and fetal blood have shown that for phenytoin the binding in the neonates and the mothers is identical, based on measurements in neonatal cord and maternal blood.[27]

Carbamazepine. Although the decreases in total plasma concentrations are not as great as for phenytoin, carbamazepine levels have been shown in a number of studies to decrease during pregnancy. Evaluation of carbamazepine is complicated by the fact that it is an active metabolite, carbamazepine 10,11-epoxide. As this metabolite has been shown to have antiepileptic effects as well as toxicity and teratogenicity, decisions regarding management of patients on carbamazepine should consider the concentrations of both the parent and the epoxide.

Carbamazepine is absorbed relatively slowly and there is wide variability in its bioavailability. This may stem from its very slow dissolution rate into the gastrointestinal fluid. Alterations of carbamazepine absorption during pregnancy have been demonstrated.

Carbamazepine distributes to lipophilic tissues such as brain and liver. Carbamazepine is rapidly distributed into the fetus.[28] It is distributed into fetal liver and kidney, but in contrast to adults, the brain concentrations are low in the fetus.

The primary metabolic pathway of carbamazepine is formation of the 10,11-epoxide. In one study of 17 patients on carbamazepine monotherapy during pregnancy, a decrease in concentration was noted throughout pregnancy.[24] This decrease was not as marked as the one observed for phenytoin.

Carbamazepine is approximately 75% protein bound, 25% unbound. No significant changes of carbamazepine binding during pregnancy have been reported.

Valproate. Decreased concentrations during pregnancy have been noted. In one study, the concentration of valproate by the third trimester was found to have fallen to less than one half of the first trimester value.

Valproate is available clinically in two basic forms: the acid form, valproic acid, and various salts, including magnesium and sodium. The acid is very quickly absorbed from the stomach, whereas the salts are generally absorbed in the small intestine. Absorption is usually complete because valproate is quite water soluble. There is no evidence that valproate absorption is affected by pregnancy.

Valproate is readily distributed to all tissues. It is present in high concentrations in blood, liver, and kidney and it distributes rapidly to the fetus.

Valproate is metabolized to a number of compounds, with the two main metabolites being 2-ene and the 3-keto. There is some suggestion that during pregnancy, valproate metabolism may be significantly altered. There is an increased clearance of valproate during the third trimester, which may have multiple mechanisms.

Valproate, like phenytoin, is highly plasma protein bound.[29] Its plasma protein binding is significantly decreased in pregnant women. In one in vitro study, the unbound fraction of the drug was found to be 14.6% in 10 women during late pregnancy, compared to 9.4% in age-matched female controls. Further complicating this phenomenon is the fact that plasma protein binding of valproate is concentration dependent, with the free fraction increasing at higher serum concentrations. Valproate readily crosses the placenta. Concentrations have been found to be higher in the placenta and umbilical cord blood than in maternal serum samples. The fetal/maternal concentration ratio has been reported to be between 1.2 to 3.0, with a mean of 1.7. The neonatal metabolism was measured with a mean half-life of 47 hours, which is much longer than the 8- to 15-hour half-lives observed in adults.

Phenobarbital and Primidone. In almost all studies, phenobarbital concentrations have been reported to be lower during pregnancy. The changes, however, are not as great as those for phenytoin and are approximately the same as for carbamazepine.[24]

Primidone is metabolized to phenobarbital as well as to phenylethylmalonamide (PEMA). Studies, though small in number, indicate that pregnancy affects primidone metabolism in a fashion similar to that of phenobarbital. Fetal metabolism of phenobarbital has been shown to be present. However, it is doubtful that it exists in a high enough degree to significantly influence the overall serum concentrations in the mother.

Newer Antiepileptic Drugs

Although few studies have been done in pregnant women, we can make several assumptions about the pharmacokinetics of the newer antiepileptic drugs.

Gabapentin is absorbed by an amino acid transport mechanism in the intestine, and pregnancy is unlikely to affect this process. Also, because gabapentin is renally eliminated, and not bound to protein, its concentrations would not be affected by changes in maternal hepatic or fetal placental metabolism or by changes in protein binding.

Lamotrigine absorption may not be affected, but its major elimination pathway is glucuronidation, and studies are needed to determine the effects of pregnancy on its concentrations.

Birth Control

Many studies have shown that doses of oral contraceptives must be increased when women are taking drugs that induce hepatic metabolism of hormones. Of the drugs used to treat epilepsy, the barbiturates, phenytoin, carbamazepine, and valproate, in that order, have the strongest inductive effect. Ethosuximide, gabapentin, and lamotrigine have the least effect.

Labor and Delivery

A frequent problem encountered during labor and delivery is increased tendency for bleeding in the neonate. This can be overcome by the use of vitamin K. The mechanism for this deficit is thought to be the induction of hepatic enzymes by antiepileptic drugs. In general, infant mortality is slightly higher in children born to epileptic mothers than to controls.[5] Vitamin D levels may often be below normal. Interestingly, neonatal jaundice seldom occurs in children exposed to antiepileptic drugs in utero, possibly because of fetal liver enzyme induction. Bone mineralization does not appear to be different in children born to mothers receiving antiepileptic drugs.

Complications of labor and delivery—such as preeclampsia, abruptio placentae, polyhydramnios, assisted delivery, cesarean section, prematurity, and intrauterine growth retardation—may be increased slightly in women with epilepsy.[5]

Drug Treatment During Pregnancy

There is no consensus about the clinical course that should be followed for pregnant epileptic women. My preference is

Table 3: FDA Classification of Antiepileptic Drugs

Schedule C drugs have no significant animal teratogenicity, but human data are limited. Schedule D drugs have both animal and human teratogenicity and should be used with caution.

Schedule C	Schedule D
gabapentin	carbamazepine
lamotrigine	valproate
levetiracetam	
tiagabine	
topiramate	

maintaining stable antiepileptic drug levels throughout pregnancy to prevent seizures from occurring. However, some women do not experience an increase in seizure frequency despite decreased antiepileptic drug levels, and some evidence suggests that teratogenicity may be related to drug concentrations. Concentrations of antiepileptic drugs should be measured at least each trimester. Blood should be drawn at each breakthrough seizure to determine whether the threshold has changed (ie, concentrations are as expected) or if there has been a change in clearance or compliance. Assuring compliance is the most important reason for obtaining antiepileptic drug levels during pregancy.[30]

Status epilepticus during pregnancy may occur in a woman with epilepsy whose seizures accelerate, or may represent a new onset of seizures in a woman with no history of epilepsy. Loading with fosphenytoin, which is rapidly converted to phenytoin, may now be the best treatment available, given at a dose of 20 mg/kg of phenytoin equivalent.[31] Fosphenytoin may replace phenytoin for loading because of its safety. If this is not effective, intravenous phenobarbital in a dose of 10 to 20 mg may be used. Diazepam has too short of a central nervous system half-life to be effective for more than one convulsion. Because status epilepticus in a patient with no history of seizures has a high probability of being caused by a brain lesion such as tumor, arteriovenous malformation, or other condition, MRI scanning should not be delayed until after delivery. A recent study has shown that magnesium sulfate may be a better treatment for seizures associated with eclampsia.[31] However, phenytoin may be needed if longer protection is needed.

Infant Care

Breast-feeding has been an issue of great concern among pregnant epileptic women. Nearly all antiepileptic drugs are transferred in breast milk. The milk concentration to serum concentration for phenytoin is 18%, for phenobarbital 36%, primidone 70%, carbamazepine 41%,[32] and only 4% to 5% for valproate.

The problem of drug effects on breast-feeding is compounded by the fact that half-lives for drugs may be increased in the neonatal period. However, only for phenobarbital and primidone have feeding difficulties and decreased weight gain been definitely correlated with maternal drug ingestion. Conversely, abrupt withdrawal of antiepileptic drugs has been thought to be a factor in isolated cases of neonatal convulsions.

Mothers with seizures can breast-feed and are able to care for their infants. However, they should take precautions when performing some tasks, such as having another person available during bathing of the infant.

Treatment of the Woman With Epilepsy During Childbearing Years

Women of childbearing potential who wish to avoid pregnancy should be counseled about the possible interactions between oral contraceptives and AEDs. Generally, the use of oral contraceptives does not exacerbate seizures, but AEDs that induce hepatic metabolism may diminish the effectiveness of oral contraceptives.[33]

Although women with epilepsy face greater risks than women with no chronic illnesses, these risks are not great enough, with a few exceptions, to preclude pregnancy. The woman and her partner have the responsibility of deciding whether to bear children. The physician's role should focus on providing information about the risks of childbearing and on providing medical care to reduce the risks as much as possible before the patient becomes pregnant. Often overlooked in this are risk factors other than epilepsy that may have much greater consequence on pregnancy than seizures or antiepi-

Table 4: Recommendations for Managing Women With Epilepsy Who Wish to Become Pregnant

Before Conception

- Educate the family regarding risks
- Review classification of epilepsy
- Determine most appropriate medicine for seizure control
- Determine need for continued medication
  - may discontinue if seizure-free for 2 or more years
  - do not discontinue medication if epilepsy syndrome suggests continued need for treatment
- Reduce medicines to monotherapy
- Start folic acid
- Eliminate other risk factors—smoking, drugs, alcohol

After Conception

- Do not change antiepileptic medication
- Refer for prenatal care
- Prescribe vitamins, including folic acid
- Check blood levels every trimester and change doses as needed
- Evaluate for neural tube defects at 12 to 16 weeks (ultrasound, alpha-fetoprotein, amniocentesis)
- Consider vitamin K predelivery
- Check antiepileptic drug levels prior to delivery and increase doses if needed

After Delivery

- Check levels
- Examine infant

leptic drugs. These risk factors are, to list a few, advancing maternal age, heavy smoking, substance abuse (alcohol, street drugs), folic acid deficiency, other prescription drugs, inadequate prenatal care, and genetic factors.

The most critical step in caring for an epileptic woman of childbearing age is to properly diagnose the syndrome. An accurate diagnosis is essential because a substantial number of women diagnosed as having intractable epilepsy in fact have experienced nonepileptic events (pseudoseizures), and therefore can avoid the risks posed by antiepileptic medications and convulsions.

Antiepileptic medications can be discontinued in some women whose seizures have been well controlled. But attempts to withdraw medications should be made well in advance of contemplated pregnancy.

Summary

All of the standard AEDs carry some risks of teratogenicity, although the newer AEDs may carry a lower risk (Table 3). In general, if an antiepileptic drug has been effective before pregnancy and its use has been carefully reviewed, there is no need to change to another drug before or during pregnancy. Generalized tonic-clonic seizures occurring during pregnancy appear to be more dangerous to the fetus than the risks posed by antiepileptic drug therapy.

Carbamazepine, phenytoin, and valproate are the most widely used drugs for partial seizures, and no study has demonstrated these drugs to differ in terms of their ability to control seizures. Phenobarbital and primidone appear to have more side effects than most others. Treatment with carbamazepine or phenytoin appears to be the most reasonable course of action once it has been determined that a pregnant woman has localization-related epilepsy and is at risk for having seizures. Women with idiopathic generalized tonic-clonic seizures or juvenile myoclonic epilepsy should be treated with valproate or lamotrigine. Pregnant women on valproate should be warned of the potential for neural tube defects. Although animal studies show that felbamate, gabapentin, levetiracetam, and lamotrigine are not associated with significant malformations, human experience is limited.

Whatever the case, quality prenatal care must be provided. Folic acid supplements of 0.8 to 5 mg/day may lower the incidence of malformations.[11] Vitamin K supplementation may be necessary to reduce bleeding problems during labor and delivery.

With optimal care (Table 4), both the patient and physician can expect a favorable outcome of pregnancy in the vast majority of instances. Consequently, epilepsy should not preclude a woman from bearing and rearing children. A practice parameter for management of women with epilepsy has been jointly developed by the American Academy of Neurology, the American Epilepsy Society, the Epilepsy Foundation of America, and the Child Neurology Society.[34]

References

1. Stanley FJ, Prescott PK, Johnston R, et al: Congenital malformations in infants of mothers with diabetes and epilepsy in Western Australia, 1980-1982. *Med J Aust* 1985;143:440-442.

2. Bjerkedal T: Outcome of pregnancy in women with epilepsy, Norway 1967 to 1978: Congenital malformations. In: Janz D, Bossi L, Dam M, et al, eds. *Epilepsy, Pregnancy, and the Child*. New York, Raven Press, 1982, pp 289-295.

3. Knight AH, Rhind EG: Epilepsy and pregnancy: a study of 153 pregnancies in 59 patients. *Epilepsia* 1975;16:99-110.

4. Schmidt D: The effect of pregnancy on the natural history of epilepsy: Review of the literature. In: Janz D, Bossi L, Dam M, et al, eds. *Epilepsy, Pregnancy, and the Child*. New York, Raven Press, 1982, pp 3-14.

5. Teramo K, Hiilesmaa VK: Pregnancy and fetal complications in epileptic pregnancies: Review of the literature. In: Janz D, Bossi L, Dam M, et al, eds. *Epilepsy, Pregnancy, and the Child*. New York, Raven Press, 1982, pp 53-59.

6. Otani K: Risk factors for the increased seizure frequency during pregnancy and puerperium. *Folia Psychiatr Neurol Jpn* 1985;39(1):33-41.

7. Schmidt D, Canger R, Avanzini G, et al: Change of seizure frequency in pregnant epileptic women. *J Neurol Neurosurg Psychiatry* 1983;46(8):751-755.

8. Minkoff H, Schaffer RM, Delke I, et al: Diagnosis of intracranial hemorrhage in utero after a maternal seizure. *Obstet Gynecol* 1985; 22S-24S.

9. Teramo K, Hiilesmaa VK, Bardy A, et al: Fetal heart rate during a maternal grand mal epileptic seizure. *J Perinat Med* 1979;7:3-6.

10. Nelson KB, Ellenberg JH: Maternal seizure disorder, outcome of pregnancy, and neurologic abnormalities in children. *Neurology* 1982;32(11):1247-1254.

11. Dansky L, Andermann E, Rosenblatt D, et al: Anticonvulsants, folate levels, and pregnancy outcome: a prospective study. *Ann Neurol* 1987; 21:176-182.

12. Friis ML, Hauge M: Congenital heart defects in live-born children of epileptic patients. *Arch Neurol* 1985;42:374-376.

13. Samrén E, Van Duijn C, Christiaens G, et al: Antiepileptic drug regimens and major congenital abnormalities in the offspring. *Ann Neurol* 1999;46(5):739-746.

14. Granstrom ML, Hiilesmaa VK: Malformations and minor anomalies in the children of epileptic mothers: preliminary results of pro-

spective Helsinki study. In: Janz D, Bossi L, Dam M, et al, eds. *Epilepsy, Pregnancy and the Child.* New York, Raven Press, 1982, pp 303-307.

15. Hanson JW, Myrianthopoulos NC, Sedgwick-Harvey MA, et al: Risks of the offspring of women treated with hydantoin anticonvulsants with emphasis on the fetal hydantoin syndrome. *J Pediatr* 1976;89:662-668.

16. Seip M: Growth retardation dysmorphic facies and minor malformations following massive exposure to phenobarbital in utero. *Acta Paediatr Scand* 1976;65:617-621.

17. Robert E, Giubaud P: Maternal valproic acid and congenital neural tube defects. *Lancet* 1982;2:937.

18. Robert E, Robert JM, Lapras C: L'acide valproique est-il teratogene? *Rev Neurol* 1983;139:445-447.

19. Rosa FW: Spina bifida infants of women treated with carbamazepine during pregnancy. *N Engl J Med* 1991;324:674-677.

20. Myhre SA, Williams R: Teratogenic effects associated with maternal primidone therapy. *J Pediatr* 1981;99(1):160-162.

21. Nakane Y, Okuma T, Takahaski R, et al: Multi-institutional study of the teratogenicity and fetal toxicity of antiepileptic drugs: a report of a collaborative study group in Japan. *Epilepsia* 1980;21(6):663-680.

22. Biale Y, Lewenthal H: Effect of folic acid supplementation on congenital malformations due to anticonvulsant drugs. *Eur J Obstet Gynecol Reprod Biol* 1984;18:211-216.

23. McElnay JC: Interaction of phenytoin with antacid constituents and kaolin. *Br J Pharmacol* 1981;70:126-127.

24. Bardy AH, Teramo K, Hiilesmaa VK: Apparent plasma clearances of phenytoin, phenobarbital, primidone, and carbamazepine during pregnancy: results of a prospective Helsinki study. In: Janz D, Bossi L, Dam M, et al, eds. *Epilepsy, Pregnancy and the Child.* New York, Raven Press, 1982, pp 141-145.

25. Stock B, Dean M, Levy G: Serum protein binding of drugs during and after pregnancy in rats. *J Pharmacol Exp Ther* 1979;212(2):264-268.

26. Dean M, Stock B, Patterson RJ, et al: Serum protein binding of drugs during and after pregnancy in humans. *Clin Pharmacol Ther* 1980;28:253-261.

27. Friel P, Yerby M, McCormick K: Use of unbound drug concentrations to determine neonatal anticonvulsant exposure. *Epilepsy Res* 1987;1:70-73.

28. Pynnonen S, Kanto J, Sillanpaa M, et al: Carbamazepine: placental transport, tissue concentrations in fetus and newborn, and level of milk. *Acta Pharmacol Toxicol* 1977;41:244-253.

29. Riva R, Albani F, Contin M, et al: Mechanism of altered drug binding to serum proteins in pregnant women: studies with valproic acid. *Ther Drug Monit* 1984;6:25-30.

30. Leppik IE, Cloyd JC, Sawchuk RJ, et al: Compliance and variability of plasma phenytoin levels in epileptic patients. *Ther Drug Monit* 1979;1:475-483.

31. Lucas MJ, Leveno KJ, Cunningham FC: A comparison of magnesium sulfate with phenytoin for the prevention of eclampsia. *N Engl J Med* 1995; 333:201-205.

32. Kaneko S, Suzuki K, Sato T, et al: The problems of antiepileptic medication in the neonatal period: Is breast-feeding advisable? In: Janz D, Bossi L, Dam M, et al, eds. *Epilepsy, Pregnancy, and the Child.* New York, Raven Press, 1982, pp 343-348.

33. Leppik E, Wolff D, Purves S: Treatment of epilepsy in women of childbearing potential; issues in management. *CNS Drugs* 1999;11(3):191-206.

34. Practice parameter: management issues for women with epilepsy (summary statement). Report of the Quality Standards Subcommittee of the American Academy of Neurology. *Neurology* 1998;51(4): 944-948.

Chapter 11

Epilepsy in the Elderly

The incidence of a first seizure is 52 to 59 per 100,000 in persons 40 to 59 years of age, but rises to 127 per 100,000 in those 60 and over.[1] Among persons 65 years and older, the active epilepsy prevalence rate is approximately 1.5%, about twice the rate of younger adults. As the elderly population continues to grow steadily, increasing numbers of them are likely to receive antiepileptic drugs (AEDs). In the elderly, the most common identifiable cause of epilepsy is stroke. Brain tumor, head injury, and Alzheimer's disease are other major causes. However, in a large number of cases, the precise cause cannot be identified.

Many physicians begin treatment after a single seizure in elderly patients because the occurrence of a second seizure is high if a lesion in the central nervous system (eg, tumor, stroke, AVM) is present. Treatment in the elderly carries more risks than in younger persons because the elderly may experience more side effects and they have a greater risk for drug interactions. In additon, they may be less able to afford the cost of medications.

Assessment of AED treatment efficacy and toxicity in elderly patients is challenging because seizures are sometimes difficult to observe, signs and symptoms of toxicity can be attributed to other causes (eg, Alzheimer's disease, stroke, etc) or to co-medications, and patients may not be able to accurately self-report problems.

In addition to their use in epilepsy, AEDs are prescribed for a variety of other neuropsychiatric disorders, including neuralgias, aggressive behavior disorders, essential tremor, and restless legs syndrome—conditions prevalent in the elderly. Treatment of older patients with AEDs, as with many other medications, is complicated by increased sensitivity to drug effects, narrow therapeutic ranges, complex pharmacokinetics, and the increased likelihood of drug interactions because of multiple drug therapy. When clinicians prescribe for the elderly, they must also consider the likelihood of concomitant disorders and the high individual variability found in this population. As a cause of adverse reactions among the elderly, AEDs rank fifth among all drug categories.[2]

In a review of 45,405 people 65 years or older living throughout the country in long-term care facilities serviced by Pharmacy Corporation of America, at least one AED was taken by 4,573 (10.1%) of the residents. Approximately 1.5 million elderly people reside in nursing homes; thus, as many as 150,000 nursing home elderly may be taking AEDs.[3]

Clinical Pharmacology of AEDs in the Elderly

The age-related physiologic changes that appear to have the greatest effect on AED pharmacokinetics are the concentration of certain serum proteins and the reduction in liver volume and blood flow. The unbound drug concentration in serum is in direct equilibrium with the concentration at the site of action and provides the best correlation with drug response.[4]

By age 65, many individuals have low normal albumin concentrations or are frankly hypoalbuminemic. Albumin concentration may be further reduced by conditions such as malnutrition, renal insufficiency, and rheumatoid arthritis. As serum albumin levels decline, drug binding will decrease. This has the effect of lowering the total serum drug concentration for phenytoin and valproate while the unbound serum drug concentration remains unchanged.

The concentration of α1-acid glycoprotein (AAG), a reactant serum protein, increases with age; further elevations occur during pathophysiologic stress such as stroke, heart failure, trauma, infection, myocardial infarction, surgery, and chronic obstructive pulmonary disease. Administration of enzyme-inducing AEDs also increases AAG. When the concentration of AAG rises, the binding of weakly alkaline and neutral drugs such as carbamazepine (and its epoxide metabolite) to AAG can increase, causing higher total serum drug and metabolite concentrations in the face of low unbound concentrations.

The total clearance of the major AEDs, which are eliminated by the liver, is primarily influenced by the extent of protein binding and intrinsic metabolizing capacity (intrinsic clearance) of unbound drug. Because total clearance determines steady-drug concentrations, age-related alterations in protein binding or intrinsic clearance can affect serum drug concentrations. Age-related reductions in intrinsic clearance result in a rise in unbound serum drug concentrations. Age-related changes in protein binding and intrinsic clearance can have variable effects on drugs and their active metabolites. For example, elimination of an active metabolite may be significantly reduced, resulting in an increase in unbound metabolite concentrations, while elimination of the parent drug remains unchanged. In this case, response to drug therapy may change, although the concentration of the parent drug, either total or unbound, remains stable.

Because of the complexity of confounding variables and the lack of correlation between simple measures of liver function and drug metabolism, the effect of age on hepatic drug metabolism remains largely unknown. Phase I reactions (oxidation, reduction, and hydroxylation) are affected to a greater extent than phase II reactions (glucuronidation, acetylation, and sulfation). For example, advanced age has little effect on the clearance of lorazepam, which undergoes glucuronidation; however, clearance of diazepam and its active metabolite, both of which undergo oxidative metabolism, are reduced.

Despite the theoretical effects of age-related physiologic changes on drug disposition and the widespread use of AEDs in the elderly, few studies on AED pharmacokinetics in the elderly have been performed. The available reports generally involve single-dose evaluations in small samples of the young old, that is, persons 65 to 74 years old. The absence of data on AED pharmacokinetics in the oldest old increases the possibility of therapeutic failure and adverse reactions in this population.

Phenytoin

Phenytoin has a narrow therapeutic range and complex pharmacokinetics. It is absorbed slowly, is approximately 90% bound to serum albumin, and undergoes saturable metabolism, which has the effect of producing nonlinear changes in steady-state serum concentrations.

Clinical studies in elderly patients have shown decreases in phenytoin binding to albumin and increases in the free fraction. The binding of phenytoin to serum proteins correlates with the albumin concentration, which is typically low normal to subnormal in the elderly. As the drug concentration rises and the albumin concentration falls, phenytoin binding is likely to decrease.

One study compared the pharmacokinetics of phenytoin at steady state after oral administration in 34 elderly (60 to 79 years), 32 middle-aged (40 to 59 years), and 26 younger adults (20 to 39 years) with epilepsy. All subjects had normal albumin concentrations and liver function and received no other medications, including other AEDs known to alter hepatic metabolism. The maximum rate of metabolism (V_{max}) declined gradually with age, and significantly lower values were seen in the elderly group compared to younger adults.[5] The smaller V_{max} means that phenytoin metabolism becomes saturated at lower concentrations than in younger patients. Thus, smaller maintenance doses of phenytoin are needed to attain desired unbound serum concentrations, and relatively small changes in dose ($\leq 10\%$) are recommended when making dosing adjustments. Thus, in the elderly, a daily dose of 3 mg/kg appears to be appropriate, rather than the 5 mg/kg per day used in younger adults. This 3 mg/kg dose is only 160 mg/day for a 52-kg woman, or 200 mg/day for a 66-kg man.

One nursing home survey revealed that residents were taking phenytoin doses similar to those used in younger adults.[6] Thus, there is a great potential for inadvertent overdose in the nursing home population. Because of protein binding, the total levels in these persons may appear to be normal, but the free (unbound level) may detect overdoses.

In patients with both reduced metabolism and binding to serum albumin, unbound concentration increases while the total drug concentration decreases. In such cases, the clinician may find that the total drug concentration does not correlate with response. Patients may achieve seizure control with what is thought to be subtherapeutic concentrations, or they may experience toxicity when total serum concentrations are in the therapeutic range. Measurement of unbound phenytoin concentrations is necessary for elderly patients who have: (1) decreased serum albumin concentration or total phenytoin concentrations that are near the upper boundary of the therapeutic range; (2) total concentrations that decline over time; (3) a low total concentration relative to the daily dose; or (4) total concentrations that do not correlate with clinical response. A range of 5 mg/L to 15 mg/L total may be more appropriate as a therapeutic range for the elderly.

Valproic Acid

Only a few small studies have compared the pharmacokinetics of valproic acid in young and old patients. In a study of steady-state valproate pharmacokinetics in 6 young adult and 6 elderly volunteers (66 to 72 years), the average unbound fraction of valproate was 10.7% in the elderly compared with 6.4% in younger subjects. In elderly subjects, mean unbound concentration was 67% higher and unbound clearance was 65% lower than in younger adults.[7] In another study comparing single-dose intravenous valproate pharmacokinetics in 7 young adult volunteers and 6 residents of long-term care units (75 to 87 years), total clearance was similar in the two groups. Serum elimination half-life was twice as long in the elderly as in the younger subjects, 14.9 vs 7.2 hours.[8] Valproic acid, like phenytoin, is associated with reduced protein binding and unbound clearance in the elderly. As a result, the desired clinical response may be achieved with a lower dose than usual. Because the serum elimination half-life is prolonged, the dosing interval can be extended. If the albumin concentration has fallen or the patient's clinical response does not correlate with total drug concentration, measurement of unbound drug should be considered.

Carbamazepine

Young adults typically require 10 to 20 mg/kg/day taken in three or four divided doses to attain serum carbamazepine concentrations within the usual therapeutic range. Carbamazepine doses were much lower in our nursing home study while trough serum carbamazepine concentrations remained within the usual therapeutic range. We calculated carbamazepine clearance in 7 residents (mean age = 82.3 years) using daily dose and trough serum concentrations. Clearance was 40% lower than in a group of younger patients, 41.0 ± 19.6 vs 71.4 ± 35.8 mL/h/kg, respectively. This decrease is the same magnitude as seen with phenytoin and valproic acid in elderly patients. The smaller clearance results in a prolonged elimination half-life. These changes in carbamazepine pharmacokinetics require lower dosages and less frequent dosing in elderly patients.

Benzodiazepines

Benzodiazepines used for the treatment of epilepsy include diazepam, lorazepam, clorazepate, and clonazepam. Diazepam and lorazepam are administered intravenously for the acute treatment of status epilepticus, and clorazepate and clonazepam are given orally as maintenance therapy.

Diazepam is highly protein bound (>99%) and undergoes oxidative metabolism to form an active metabolite, desmethyldiazepam. Protein binding declines with age, resulting in an increased free fraction and a greater distribution volume of diazepam and desmethyldiazepam. Unbound clearance is reduced, prolonging the serum elimination half-life of the drug and its metabolite. Lorazepam is less highly bound (90%) and is metabolized by conjugation to lorazepam glucuronide. The free fraction of lorazepam rises with age, and the volume of distribution is increased, but less than with diazepam. The elimination half-life of lorazepam is similar in the young and the elderly. Direct comparisons of the pharmacokinetics of clonazepam and clorazepate in the young and the elderly have not been published.

The elderly tend to be more sensitive to drugs that act on the central nervous system. Among such drugs, the benzodiazepines have undergone the most extensive pharmacodynamic investigation. In a study of diazepam sedation, sensitivity was increased in the elderly, although unbound drug concentrations did not differ from those in younger subjects.[9] The increased sensitivity of the elderly to such drugs is apparently independent of drug concentration, either in the serum or at the site of action. The enhanced sensitivity of the elderly to benzodiazepines may extend to other AEDs as well.

Drug Interactions

Concomitant medications taken by elderly patients can alter the absorption, distribution, and metabolism of AEDs, thereby increasing the risk of toxicity or therapeutic failure. For example, calcium-containing antacids and sucralfate reduce the absorption of phenytoin. The absorption of phenytoin, carbamazepine, and valproate may be reduced significantly by oral antineoplastic drugs that damage gastrointestinal cells. In addition, phenytoin concentrations may be lowered by intravenously administered antineoplastic agents. The use of folic acid for treatment of megaloblastic anemia may decrease serum concentrations of phenytoin, and enteral feedings can also lower serum concentrations in patients receiving orally administered phenytoin.[10]

Many drugs displace AEDs from plasma proteins, an effect that is especially serious when the interacting drug also inhibits the metabolism of the displaced drug; this occurs when valproate interacts with phenytoin. Several drugs used on a short-term basis (including propoxyphene and erythromycin) or as maintenance therapy (such as cimetidine, diltiazem, fluoxetine, and verapamil) significantly inhibit the metabolism of one or more AEDs by the P-450 system. Certain agents can induce the P-450 system or other enzymes, causing an increase in drug metabolism. The most commonly prescribed inducers of drug metabolism are phenytoin, phenobarbital, and carbamazepine. Ethanol, when used chronically, also induces drug metabolism. The interaction between antipsychotic drugs and AEDs is complex. Hepatic metabolism of certain antipsychotics such as haloperidol can be increased by carbamazepine, resulting in diminished psychotropic response. Antipsychotic medications, especially chlorpromazine, promazine, trifluoperazine, and perphenazine, can reduce the threshold for seizures. The risk of seizures is directly proportional to the total number of psychotropic medications being taken, their doses, any abrupt increases in doses, and the presence of organized brain pathology. The epileptic patient taking antipsychotic drugs may need a higher dose of antiepileptic medication to control seizures. In contrast, central nervous system depressants are likely to lower the maximum dose of AEDs that can be administered before toxic symptoms occur.

References

1. Hauser WA, Hesdorffer DC, eds: *Epilepsy. Frequency, Causes and Consequences.* New York, NY, Demos Publications, 1990, pp 1-51.

2. Moore SA, Teal TW, eds: Adverse drug reaction surveillance in the geriatric population: a preliminary review. *Proceedings of the Drug Information Association Workshop Geriatric Drug Use: Clinical and Social Perspectives.* Washington, DC, Pergamon Press, 1985.

3. Lackner T, Cloyd J, Thomas L, et al: Antiepileptic drug use in nursing home residents: effect of age, gender, comedication on patterns of use. *Epilepsy* 1998;39(10):1083-1087.

4. Wallace SM, Verbeeck RK: Plasma protein binding of drugs in the elderly. *Clin Pharmacokinet* 1987;12:41-72.

5. Bauer LA, Blouin RA: Age and phenytoin kinetics in adult epileptics. *Clin Pharmacol Ther* 1982;31:301-304.

6. Cloyd J, Lackner T, Leppik I: Antiepileptics in the elderly. *Arch Fam Med* 1994;3:589-598.

7. Bauer LA, Davis R, Wilensky A, et al: Valproic acid clearance: unbound fraction and diurnal variation in young and elderly adults. *Clin Pharmacol Ther* 1985;37:697-700.

8. Bryson SM, Verma N, Scott PJW, et al: Pharmacokinetics of valproic acid in young and elderly subjects. *Br J Clin Pharmacol* 1983;16:104-105.

9. Cook PJ, Flanagan R, James IM: Diazepam tolerance: effect of age, regular sedation and alcohol. *Br Med J* 1984;289:351-353.

10. Haley CJ, Nelson J: Phenytoin-enteral feeding interaction. *Ann Pharmacother* 1989;23:796-798.

Chapter 12

Acute Repetitive Seizures and Status Epilepticus

The classical definition of status epilepticus (SE) is a condition characterized by an epileptic seizure that is so frequently repeated or so prolonged as to create a fixed and lasting condition.[1] SE is actually at the extreme of a continuum of seizure frequencies (Figure 1). Status epilepticus is a medical emergency that requires prompt and appropriate treatment. Any type of epileptic seizure can develop into SE. The syndrome most commonly associated with SE is tonic-clonic (convulsive) status epilepticus; an estimated 60,000 to 150,000 persons in the United States will have at least one episode of convulsive SE in a given year. Recently, nonconvulsive SE has been recognized as a cause of unresponsiveness or coma in as many as 8% of hospitalized persons. It is important to obtain an EEG in anyone with unexplained stupor or coma.[2]

However, animal studies and clinical experience have shown that each seizure may predispose the brain to additional, harder-to-control seizures. Therefore, emergency treatment to prevent SE is more appropriate than delaying therapy until all of the criteria of the classic definition have been met.

In convulsive SE, the patient suffers from repeated generalized tonic-clonic (GTC) seizures without recovering consciousness and remains in the postictal state between seizures. Generalized tonic-clonic seizures usually last for 2 to 3 minutes, during which the patient convulses violently. Because of the tonic axial muscle contraction, respiration is halted. During the clonic phase, small amounts of air may be exchanged. The patient often appears cyanotic because of desaturation of the hemoglobin and because of increased intrathoracic pressure impeding venous return. Immediately after the GTC seizure, respiratory drive increases and the patient has deep, rapid respiration. If the SE is not caused by an acute central nervous system (CNS) insult, the level of consciousness may increase before the next seizure; but if there is no improve-

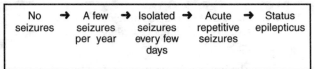

| No seizures | → | A few seizures per year | → | Isolated seizures every few days | → | Acute repetitive seizures | → | Status epilepticus |

Figure 1—*The continuum of seizures frequency.*

ment in consciousness, a new CNS insult should be suspected (Table 1, Group II).

In adults with SE, GTC seizures are usually followed by 20 to 30 minutes of the postictal state, which is then followed by another seizure. In children, GTC seizures may be continuous. Repeated GTC seizures can lead to systemic cardiovascular dysfunction. The cardiovascular system is particularly stressed from the excessive demands placed on it by the repeated tonic contractions of the skeletal muscle system. Tachycardia is inevitable; bradycardia may occur from vagal tone modulated by CNS activity; and cardiac arrhythmias may occur from hyperkalemia. Drugs used to treat SE may contribute to these problems; barbiturates may depress the myocardium, and phenytoin and its solvent, propylene glycol, may cause arrhythmias and hypotension.

While a single GTC seizure is usually followed by great respiratory effort stimulated by hypercarbia, respiratory failure may occur after a series of seizures. The disorder that precipitates SE can itself depress respiratory drive, as can barbiturates and benzodiazepines used to treat the patient. Altered lymph flow may induce pulmonary edema. Rhabdomyolysis leads to myoglobinuria and may cause renal failure. The metabolic-biochemical complications of GTC seizures include respiratory and metabolic acidosis, anoxemia, hyperazotemia, hyperkalemia, hypoglycemia, and hyponatremia. Massive activation of both sympathetic and parasympathetic systems leads to severe autonomic nervous system disturbances, including hyperpyrexia, excessive sweating, and salivary and tracheobronchial hypersecretion. Endocrine abnormalities—including marked elevations in plasma prolactin, in glucagon, in growth hormone, and in adrenocorticotrophic hormone (ACTH)—have been reported. There may also be cerebrospinal fluid pleocytosis attributable to SE.

Table 1: Static or Acute CNS Pathology as Causes of Status Epilepticus*

Group I - Static

- Exacerbation of seizures in patients with epilepsy
- Alcohol or drug abuse
- Withdrawal from drugs
- Miscellaneous or undetermined (no acute CNS lesion or metabolic cause identified)

Group II - Acute

- Anoxic encephalopathy
- Acute vascular event (stroke, intercerebral hemorrhage)
- CNS neoplasm
- Acute trauma
- Metabolic encephalopathy
- Meningitis

* Modified from Cranford et al[4]

Mortality and Morbidity

Damage to the CNS may be caused by the systemic effects of the seizures described above or by prolonged electrical discharges within the brain. Prolonged electrical activity within the CNS may cause irreversible neuronal damage. Meldrum and coworkers have shown in animal models that if the abnormal electrical activity is not suppressed, neuronal damage results even when animals are paralyzed and ventilated to prevent the metabolic consequences of the convulsions.[3] The condition of nonconvulsive SE in patients is the human analog of this situation, and if not recognized and treated, can lead to significant mortality.[2]

What Causes Status Epilepticus?

The reported causes of convulsive SE vary and reflect the population served by hospitals. Two broad groups of patients can be identified (Table 1): those with no new structural CNS lesion (Group I) and those with an acute CNS injury (Group II). Group I includes patients with a history of epilepsy who have an acute exacerbation of seizures. Withdrawal from anti-epileptic drugs causes exacerbation of seizures in most of these

Table 2: Treatment to Prevent Status Epilepticus	
Initiate Treatment	• after 1 generalized tonic-clonic seizure lasting more than 5 min, or
	• after 2 generalized tonic-clonic seizures occurring in 1 hour
Use either	
Protocol A or	lorazepam 4 mg IV followed by fosphenytoin 20 mg/kg
Protocol B	fosphenytoin 20 mg/kg, using small doses of lorazepam or diazepam as needed

patients and may be documented by measuring drug serum levels. Drug abuse involving crack cocaine, amphetamines, phencyclidine (PCP, "angel dust") or other street drugs may trigger SE. Unusual causes for seizure exacerbation include baclofen withdrawal or secondary hyperparathyroidism. Prognosis for Group I patients is generally good if treatment is instituted quickly.

Group II patients are those with an acute neurologic insult, such as head injury, rapidly growing brain tumor, anoxic encephalopathy, meningitis, encephalitis, or other acute CNS process. Prognosis for Group II patients is usually poor. They often have seizures after phenytoin loading and often need phenobarbital loading. If this is ineffective, they may need phenobarbital coma. Mortality rates may be as high as 33%,[4] but in most cases, mortality can be attributed to the condition that caused the Group II SE, ie, anoxic encephalopathy.

Not all patients appearing to have continuous seizures are having convulsive status epilepticus. The syndrome of nonepileptic SE, in which a person has serial nonepileptic convulsions (pseudoseizures), must be considered whenever there is an unusual presentation for the seizure type or if response to antiepileptic drugs does not follow the expected pattern. Occasionally, a person with intermittent decorticate or decerebrate posturing may be mistakenly diagnosed as having SE.

Treatment

In the past, attention has been directed at treatment of status epilepticus. However, there is increasing experimental

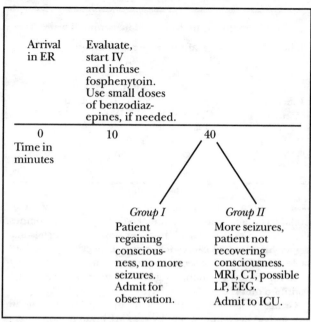

Arrival in ER	Evaluate, start IV and infuse fosphenytoin. Use small doses of benzodiazepines, if needed.	
0 Time in minutes	10	40
	Group I Patient regaining consciousness, no more seizures. Admit for observation.	*Group II* More seizures, patient not recovering consciousness. MRI, CT, possible LP, EEG. Admit to ICU.

Figure 2—Time frame for the emergency treatment of seizures and status epilepticus.

and clinical evidence to indicate that each seizure may worsen the prognosis. Thus, many physicians are developing strategies and protocols to prevent the development of SE. Some patients with severe epilepsy may develop acute repetitive seizures. These may evolve into status epilepticus and require prompt treatment. Rectal diazepam solution has been found to be an effective treatment for this condition.[5]

In adults, the vast majority of single, self-limited generalized, tonic-clonic seizures last 2 minutes, with the maximum being 4 minutes. Any seizure lasting 5 minutes or more should be treated aggressively (Table 2), rather than waiting for a seizure to last 30 minutes to meet the classical definition of SE.[1] Two or more generalized tonic-clonic seizures in an hour should also warrant aggressive treatment. More aggressive treatment is now possible with the availability of fosphenytoin

(Cerebyx®), which has greatly decreased the risks of treatment and should replace parenteral phenytoin. Parenteral phenytoin solution has 40% propylene glycol (antifreeze) and its pH is adjusted to 12 with sodium hydroxide (drain cleaner).

Time is critical in the appropriate treatment of SE. Every facility likely to treat SE should have a sequence of treatment to be instituted because it is easy for clinicians to be distracted by other pressing needs.

Figure 2 and Table 2 reflect protocols for aggressive treatment.

The first few minutes should be spent assessing the patient's overall condition. An examination should be made for clues that might indicate an etiology for the particular episode of SE. Medical alert bracelets worn by persons with epilepsy may provide helpful information. Evidence of a recent head injury may suggest the presence of an intracerebral hematoma. Historical details surrounding the onset of SE should be obtained. Such information can often be provided by paramedical personnel or by friends or relatives accompanying the patient. Diagnostic laboratory testing should be done to rule out metabolic causes of seizures. Status epilepticus from hypoglycemia, hyponatremia, and other metabolic conditions do not respond to antiepileptic medications. Drug therapy should begin as soon as it becomes clear that the patient meets the criteria for treatment. The most important clinical sign is recovery of consciousness. This is why we use benzodiazepines sparingly and only if the onset of another convulsion is heralded by low-amplitude clonic activity.

Diazepam

Diazepam became popular in the mid-1960s after a few case reports indicated its success in treating SE. Its profile of activity is a function of the drug's physiochemical properties. Because approximately 20% of cardiac output goes to the brain, as much as 20% of an intravenous dose of diazepam enters the CNS after injection, accounting for the rapid onset of anticonvulsant activity of this drug.

However, the binding of diazepam to the benzodiazepam receptor site is relatively weak. Furthermore, diazepam is also quite lipid soluble and, with recirculation, the relatively high initial brain concentrations decrease quickly as diazepam is redistributed to the greater bulk of fatty tissue. Thus, the

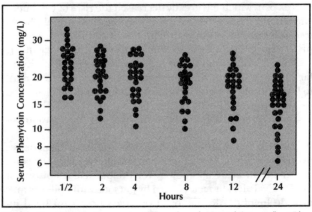

Figure 3—Serum concentrations after doses of 18 mg/kg. The patient's weight was estimated, accounting for some of the scatter. Preloading concentrations were obtained, and any patient with measurable phenytoin concentrations was excluded. Data from Cranford et al.[14] Used with permission, Neurology 1978.

duration of diazepam's effectiveness in the brain is less than 30 minutes. Its short, cerebral half-life has been demonstrated in cat models through simultaneous measurements of EEG recordings and of blood and brain concentrations.[6] A similar time course has been observed in the treatment of clinical SE when a significant number of patients receiving diazepam alone had recurrence of seizures.[4] In view of these findings, it is no longer sufficient simply to administer a dose of diazepam, return to other pressing duties, and plan for additional treatment only if seizures reoccur. Instead, diazepam should be used in conjunction with, or be followed by, loading with a medication with a longer course of action in the CNS.

Lorazepam

Lorazepam has higher affinity binding to the benzodiazepam receptor sites when compared to diazepam, and, theoretically, a longer effective life at the receptor site.

In the first double-blind, random study of benzodiazepines in SE (N = 78), a single 4-mg dose of lorazepam was com-

Table 3: Propofol Treatment of Refractory Status Epilepticus in the ICU[13]

- Loading dose: 1 mg/kg IV as slow IV bolus over 5 min, followed by a second bolus of 1 mg/kg if needed
- Maintenance: 2 to 4 mg/kg/h but may be adjusted as much as 15 mg/kg/h using EEG monitoring to attain suppression of spikes on EEG
- Use: IV fluids and low-dose dopamine to treat hypotension
- Taper infusion: every 8 to 12 h and monitor EEG. Resume maintenance for an additional 8 to 12 h if spike activity returns.

pared with a 10-mg dose of diazepam and found to be equivalent in terms of effectiveness and number of side effects.[7] Overall, one or two consecutive doses of diazepam (10 mg) or lorazepam (4 mg) were effective in 76% and 89% of 81 episodes, respectively. Depression of respiration in some patients was observed with both medications (Table 3).

Because this study[7] was double-blind and many of the subjects would receive diazepam, the protocol's safety component required that all patients be given an 18 mg/kg phenytoin load 30 minutes after the infusion of the study drug, regardless of whether seizures had occurred. Therefore, this trial could not answer the question of differences in the duration of action of the two study drugs.

At this time, lorazepam has been approved in Canada for use in SE; approval in the United States for use in SE is pending. Midazolam has been found to be useful for refractory status epilepticus. It can be given as an IV bolus of 0.2 mg/kg followed by continuous infusion of 0.00075 to 0.0011 mg/kg/min.[8] Some clinicians have also used midazolam instead of diazepam or lorazepam initially. Clonazepam has been used successfully in Europe for the treatment of SE, but a parenteral form is not available in the United States.

The role of benzodiazepines in SE is limited because they depress consciousness and respiration. These adverse effects may be critical during assessment of the level of consciousness after a series of seizures. Return of consciousness after GTC seizure is typical of a Group I patient, while no change or deepening of stupor or coma after a seizure may alert the physician that this is a Group II patient (Figure 2). In addition, since benzodiazepines depress respiratory drive, postictal monitoring of respiration is crucial after using this class of drug; the physician should therefore be ready to intubate if necessary.

Phenytoin

The main advantages of phenytoin are its effectiveness in controlling convulsions, its relatively long half-life, and its lack of significant CNS depression. Phenytoin is effective in suppressing experimental seizures as soon as adequate brain concentrations are attained, which, in rats, is within a few minutes.[9] In humans, high brain concentrations of phenytoin are achieved within 30 minutes.[10]

Phenytoin solution contains propylene glycol and has a pH of 12. Injection of a bolus of undiluted phenytoin by hand can be dangerous if given too rapidly and may cause severe cardiac distrubances. A troublesome complication of IV phenytoin is the *purple glove syndrome* in which a painful swollen hand develops after infusion into a dorsal hand vein.[11] Fosphenytoin is a much safer preparation and should be used instead of phenytoin. Unlike phenytoin, fosphenytoin (Cerebyx®) is stable for 120 days at room temperature after repackaging in plastic syringes and is compatible with a large range of IV fluids, including dextrose 5% in water, normal saline, lactated Ringers, 10% amino acid, 20% mannitol, 6% hetastarch, and 5% Plasmanate®.

Except for side effects, all of the other characteristics regarding phenytoin apply to fosphenytoin because it is fully converted to phenytoin. The dosing is identical. Fosphenytoin can be given more rapidly, at a rate up to 150 mg/min. It is also well absorbed and tolerated after IM administration.[12]

Additional treatment is necessary at this point. Arrangements should be made for diagnostic tests and intensive care, and further treatment with drugs should be instituted (Figure 1). These include use of phenobarbital, pentobarbital coma, midazolam drip, and propofol (Diprivan®). Propofol is a short-acting barbiturate.

After a dose of 18 mg/kg, most patients attain serum concentrations between 25 and 30 mg/L (Figure 3).

The volume of distribution of phenytoin in adults is 0.78 L/kg.[11] This means that a loading dose of 20 mg/kg will result in blood concentration of approximately 26 g/mL at the end of infusion (assuming the level was zero prior to the load). Depending on the patient's metabolism, these concentrations are maintained between 15 and 20 mg/L over 24 hours, and additional phenytoin need not be given. The patient's weight can be estimated, and most clinicians can guess the weight to within 15%. The half-life of phenytoin after doses of 18 to 20 mg/kg is in excess of 36 hours.[12] Thus, after one load of phenytoin, blood levels will remain high for many hours. Brain concentrations of phenytoin in humans parallel blood concentrations after 30 minutes.[9] If seizures continue after a loading dose of phenytoin, other agents should be used because the administration of more phenytoin will result in toxic levels and in possibly precipitating more seizures. The kinetics of intravenous phenytoin have not been well studied in children, but it would be expected that the volume of distribution and thus the loading dose would be similar to that in adults.

If Seizures Persist

If the seizures do not respond to phenytoin infusion, there is a high probability that a significant acute CNS insult has occurred and that the patient belongs to Group II.

Additional treatment is necessary at this point. Arrangements should be made for diagnostic tests and intensive care, and further treatment with drugs should be instituted (Figure 2). These include use of phenobarbital, pentobarbital coma, midazolam drip, and propofol (Diprivan®). Propofol is a short-acting barbiturate and is becoming the drug of choice because the time of attainment of seizure control was 2.6 minutes following propofol compared to 123 minutes for high-dose barbiturates (Table 3).[13]

Phenobarbital has the advantages of a long half-life and effectiveness in both generalized and partial seizures. It can also be administered more rapidly than phenytoin. Phenobarbital's disadvantages are that it depresses consciousness and respiration; the respiratory depression may be more profound in a patient initially treated with diazepam. Phenobarbital's volume of distribution is approximately 1, meaning that 1 mg/kg should result in a serum concentration of approximately 1 g/mL. A loading dose of approximately 10 mg/kg of phenobarbital is often used and can be followed by an additional dose of 10 mg/kg if needed. When a patient has been given a load of phenobarbital, an EEG must be obtained because the brain may continue to have electrical seizure activity in the absence of visible motor seizures. Also, patients not recovering consciousness after convulsions may be having "subtle status epilepticus" and need further clinical treatment.[15]

If a patient continues to have SE, either with only electrical discharges in the EEG or with continued motor seizures, pentobarbital coma should be instituted. This should be done in an intensive care unit (ICU) and should involve a neurologist and an anesthesiologist.

Pentobarbital coma has been successfully used in SE refractory to diazepam, phenytoin or other drugs.[16] Its use needs to be carefully monitored by EEG recording. Doses should be tailored to maintain a burst suppression pattern on the EEG (Figure 3). Treatment with pentobarbital coma may be required for many days or even weeks.

Treatment of SE in Infants and in Children

Diagnosis of SE in the neonate may be difficult because the seizures are subtle, with symptoms including sucking, random eye movements, stretching, yawning, bicycling movements of the legs, and apnea.[17] Seizures in neonates are unlike those seen in older persons because of the lack of myelin and dendritic connections. Nevertheless, these seizures are often associated with serious CNS disturbances. A standard loading dose of 20 to 25 mg/kg of phenobarbital has been found to be effective.[18] This may be followed by a dose of phenytoin, 20 mg/kg. In addition to these drugs, benzodiazepines are used by some pediatricians. Paraldehyde is useful in some instances; however, its availability is becoming limited in the United States and it may become unavailable in the future.

Nonconvulsive generalized SE consists of frequent or continuous absence seizures and is characterized clinically by clouding of consciousness. The EEG usually shows typical 3-Hz, generalized spike-and-wave discharges. Although absence status is most common in children and adolescents, it is occasionally reported in adults. Complex partial SE may present with clinical behavior ranging from a "twilight" state, with partial responsiveness and semipurposeful automatisms, to total unresponsiveness, speech arrest, and stereotypical automatisms. Aphasic SE, characterized by episodes of inability to speak that last from a few hours to several days, must be considered in patients presenting with dysphasia or aphasia with no other findings of cerebrovascular disease. Fortunately, the EEG is usually diagnostic for these conditions; treatment with benzodiazepam (during the EEG) often results in a rapid normalization of the EEG and clearing of the sensorium. The differential diagnosis of an acute confusional state should always include absence ("petit mal") SE and complex partial SE.

References

1. Gastaut H: Clinical and electroencephalographic classification of epileptic seizures. *Epilepsia* 1970;11:102-113.

2. Towne A, Waterhouse E, Boggs J: Prevalence of nonconvulsive status epilepticus in comatose patients. *Neurology* 2000;54:340-345.

3. Meldrum B: Psychological changes during prolonged seizures and epileptic brain damage. *Neuropediatrics* 1978;9:203-212.

4. Cranford RE, Leppik IE, Patrick B, et al: Intravenous phenytoin in acute treatment of seizures. *Neurology* 1979;29:1474-1479.

5. Dreifuss F, Rosman N, Cloyd J, et al: A comparison of rectal diazepam gel and placebo for acute repetitive seizures. *N Engl J Med* 1998;338:1869-1875.

6. Celesia GG, Booker HE, Sato S: Brain and serum concentrations of diazepam in experimental epilepsy. *Epilepsia* 1974;15:417-425.

7. Leppik IE, Derivan AT, Homan RW, et al: Double-blind study of lorazepam and diazepam in status epilepticus. *JAMA* 1983;249(11):1452-1454.

8. Parent JM, Lowenstein DH: Treatment of refractory generalized status epilepticus with continuous infusion of midazolam. *Neurology* 1994; 44:1837-1840.

9. Leppik IE, Sherwin AL: Intravenous phenytoin and phenobarbital: anticonvulsant action, brain content, and plasma binding in rat. *Epilepsia* 1979;20:201-217.

10. Wilder BJ, Ramsay E, Wilmore LJ, et al: Efficacy in intravenous phenytoin in the treatment of status epilepticus. *Ann Neurol* 1977;1:511-518.

11. Hanna DR: Purple glove syndrome: a complication of intravenous phenytoin. *J Neurosci Nurs* 1992;24:340-345.

12. Leppik IE, Boucher BA, Wilder BJ, et al: Pharmacokinetics and safety of phenytoin prodrug given IV or IM in patients. *Neurology* 1990;40:456-460.

13. Stecker MM, Kramer TH, Raps EC, et al: Treatment of refractory status epilepticus with propofol: clinical and pharmacokinetic findings. *Epilepsia* 1998;39(1):18-26.

14. Cranford RE, Leppik IE, Patrick B, et al: Intravenous phenytoin: clinical and pharmacokinetic aspects. *Neurology* 1978;28:874-880.

15. Treiman DM, Walton NY, Kendrick CW: A progressive sequence of electroencephalographic changes during generalized convulsive status epilepticus. *Epilepsy Res* 1990;5:49-60.

16. Lowenstein DH, Aminoff MJ, Simon RP: Barbiturate anesthesia in the treatment of status epilepticus. *Neurology* 1988;38:395-400.

17. Rothner AD, Erenberg G: Status epilepticus. *Pediatr Clin North Am* 1980;27:593-602.

18. Lockman LA, Kriel R, Laske D, et al: Phenobarbital dose for control of neonatal seizures. *Neurology* 1979;29: 1445-1449.

Chapter 13

Other Treatment Options: Surgery, Vagus Nerve Stimulator, the Ketogenic Diet

Although 70% to 80% of patients with epilepsy can maintain control of their seizures with minimal side effects, an estimated 500,000 to 800,000 patients in the United States cannot, and are considered to have intractable epilepsy.

Patients are considered to have intractable epilepsy when their seizures have not been brought under complete control within 1 year after appropriate therapy has been started and documented with blood levels.[1] The diagnostic codes for various seizure types include categories for intractable epilepsy (Table 1). Because the severity of epilepsy varies among patients, use of the categories in Table 1 is necessary to correctly code patients with epilepsy.

The goal of treatment should be complete freedom from seizures, and today this is more attainable than ever before because of more accurate diagnosis of epilepsy syndromes, rational polypharmacy, surgical intervention, and the ketogenic diet. These approaches are best performed by an epileptologist working in an epilepsy center. An epileptologist is usually a neurologist who has as his or her professional focus the treatment of epilepsy. An epilepsy center typically consists of a team of epileptologists, psychologists, neurosurgeons, nurses, technicians, and other professionals whose practice is organized around the comprehensive treatment of epilepsy.

Surgery

Surgery has begun to play a larger role in the treatment of epilepsy. The advent of improved drug therapy has contributed to the rising use of surgery because it is now possible to rapidly maximize a patient's drug treatment, using blood levels to assess optimal treatment. Animal studies have shown that repeated seizures may cause changes within the brain that may increase the probability of further seizures. Epilepsy should be controlled as soon as possible after its onset. Also, the social and emotional consequences of further seizures can be serious: loss of job, loss of driving privileges, and depression.

Table 1: ICD-9-CM Diagnostic Codes for Epilepsy

Diagnosis	Intractable	Not intractable
Generalized convulsive epilepsy	345.11	345.10
Partial epilepsy, with impairment of consciousness	345.41	345.40
Partial epilepsy, without mention of impairment of consciousness	345.51	345.50
Other forms of epilepsy	345.81	345.80
Epilepsy unspecified	345.91	345.90

Using outpatient video-EEG monitoring, MRI with special views of the temporal lobe, neuropsychological testing, and a careful history, a diagnosis of mesial temporal sclerosis can often be made. Persons with this syndrome usually have seizures poorly controlled by AEDs, but may have a very favorable outcome from surgery.

Four types of surgery are available: removal of one lobe, usually the temporal lobe (temporal lobectomy); removal of cortex (topectomy); removal of a hemisphere (hemispherectomy); and separation of the two hemispheres by cutting the corpus callosum.

By far the most widely performed surgery for epilepsy is temporal lobectomy. This is very successful in patients who have a specific epilepsy syndrome of mesial temporal sclerosis.[2] Although success rates vary from center to center, complete control of seizures has been reported in up to 75% of cases, and worthwhile improvement in up to 90%.[3] More difficult is the removal of some portion of cortex; often, intracranial recording is required before surgery to achieve precise localization of the epileptogenic region and areas of "eloquent cortex," which cannot be removed without causing damage.

Hemispherectomy is reserved for a few patients with severe damage to one hemisphere with the presence of a relatively normal contralateral hemisphere. Corpus callosotomy is useful in patients with multifocal damage with rapid spread of seizure activity from one hemisphere to the other. Although surgery is increasing, there is little likelihood that this option will be useful for most patients with epilepsy. Nevertheless, an evaluation directed at establishing the appropriateness for surgery should be done for any patient whose seizures have not come under complete control.

Surgery for epilepsy remained limited until the last decade, when great improvements in diagnosis and surgical techniques made surgery available to a large number of patients with intractable epilepsy.[4,5]

Presurgical Evaluation

The most important element in successful outcome of surgery is accurate identification of the origin of the seizure. A critical development has been the use of inpatient video-EEG recording of seizures. Patients with intractable epilepsy are admitted to special units in which their antiepileptic medications are withdrawn, while they are monitored around the clock with EEG recording. Special electrodes, such as sphenoidal electrodes inserted through the masseter muscle to lodge near the foramen ovale, can be used to record from medial temporal lobes.

Neuropsychological testing is crucial in helping identify local areas of dysfunction. For example, deficits in verbal memory implicate the left temporal lobe. Because temporal lobectomy should be avoided if the remaining temporal lobe cannot maintain memory function, the intracarotid Amytal® test (Wada's test) is critical.[6] During this test, first one and then the other carotid artery is injected with Amytal®, resulting in arrest of cerebral function of the injected area. Speech and memory testing is performed, and one is thus able to determine the approximate functional capacity of the opposite hemisphere in the absence of the injected hemisphere, providing an assessment of postoperative functioning.

Magnetic resonance imaging (MRI) has become an important diagnostic tool and has now made it possible to detect subtle hippocampal atrophy and mesial temporal sclerosis.

If all four tests give congruent evidence of unilateral temporal involvement—surface EEG, neuropsychologic testing, MRI, and Wada—it may not be necessary to perform additional tests before surgery. However, if there is suggestion of bitemporal involvement, depth electrodes may be needed. In the past, almost all patients underwent depth electrode re-

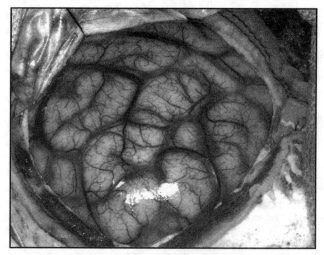

Figure 1—Placement of subdural grid for recording from the brain to locate onset of seizures. The contact points are spaced at 1-cm intervals. Stimulation is performed to map out the motor and speech areas. Above: before grid placement. Below: after grid placement.

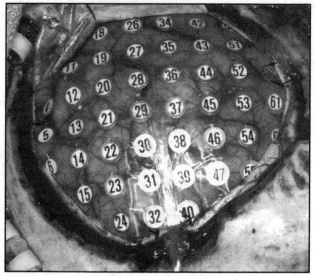

cordings prior to surgery. Positron emission tomography (PET scans) is useful in identifying focal areas of brain hypometabolism and may provide additional localizing and lateralizing information. A new development is the use of MRI for functional mapping of the brain.

Patients with frontal, parietal, and occipital lobe epilepsy are also potential surgical candidates. In these cases, however, cortical mapping before surgery may be necessary. Today, this can be done by implanting subdural grids from which stimulation and recording can be done to map the brain, much as was done by Penfield, but with the advantage of much longer recording and stimulating periods. The subdural grids may be used for 1 or 2 weeks before surgery (Figure 1). These grids are necessary in patients who have seizures emanating from the posterior part of the brain's temporal lobe in the speech-dominant hemisphere or in those where the origin is close to the motor strip.

Most surgery for epilepsy is done in the temporal lobe. However, many patients with intractable epilepsy are not good surgical candidates because of bitemporal or extratemporal foci. Some of these may be approached after grid mapping but, generally, complete remission of seizures is not as favorable, with 50% or less complete cure rates.

Some patients develop severe unihemispheral disorders, such as Rasmussen's encephalitis. Hemispherectomy may be quite helpful for these cases.[7] In patients with multifocal epilepsy with rapid generalization, cutting the corpus callosum can be useful for "drop" seizures in which patients suddenly fall to the floor, often sustaining major injuries. However, partial seizures may remain unaffected.[8]

The Vagus Nerve Stimulator

The vagus nerve stimulator (VNS) may be a treatment option for patients who have intractable epilepsy but who are not candidates for surgical options. The vagus nerve stimulator is flat, round, and about the size of a hockey puck. It contains a battery pack, a computer chip, and connecting wire.

Similar to a cardiac pacemaker, the VNS is implanted in the chest under the clavicle, and the leads at the end of the connecting wire are attached to the vagus nerve, on the left side of the neck (Figure 2). With this device, the vagus nerve can be stimulated approximately every 5 minutes for about

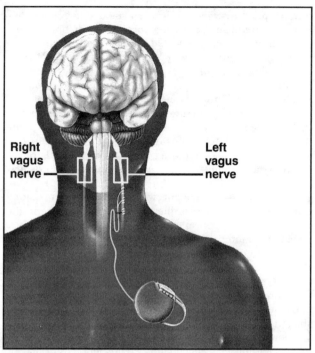

Figure 2: *The Vagus Nerve Stimulator is flat and round and is implanted in the patient's chest. The stimulating wire is wrapped around the left vagus nerve. (Note: the patient is facing you).*

30 seconds. The stimulation parameters can be adjusted by an external magnetic device controlled by a laptop computer in the physician's office. In addition, an external magnet can be applied by a caregiver during a seizure to stop the convulsion.

The vagus nerve stimulator works in animal models of epilepsy. Patients who experience *auras* warning them of an impending seizure can stop or shorten the length of the seizure by activating the VNS. This is done by holding a magnet over the pocket of skin that hides the VNS. The VNS is about as effective as the new antiepileptic drugs in reducing seizures.

Based on two double-blind studies demonstrating efficacy and safety, the Food and Drug Administration (FDA) approved the VNS for the treatment of epilepsy in 1997.

The Ketogenic Diet

The ketogenic diet is a high fat, low protein and carbohydrate diet used to treat intractable epilepsy. It was originally developed in the 1920s by scientists at the Mayo Clinic. It was widely used until after World War II when many antiepileptic medications were introduced that were generally more effective and easier to use.

However, some specialists continue to use the ketogenic diet to treat children with intractable epilepsy who do not respond to AEDs. In the early 1990s, the parents of one young patient who became seizure-free as a result of following the diet created the Charlie Foundation to Help Cure Pediatric Epilepsy. The foundation's purpose is to inform other parents and medical professionals about the ketogenic diet. Since then, the ketogenic diet has been placed on the FDA list of 'experimental treatments.'

The diet is designed to place the body into a state of starvation forcing it to use more fat than normal for energy. This results in the production of ketones—hence the name *ketogenic*.

The brain normally uses glucose manufactured from muscle tissue as its source of fuel. When the body is fasting, the brain is forced to use ketones manufactured from body fat. When this happens, the body is in a state of *ketosis*. Maintaining ketosis seems to be critical to the success of the ketogenic diet. However, the mechanism of its effect on seizures is unknown.

The ketogenic diet holds promise for some patients, particularly children, who endure multiple daily seizures that can not be controlled by any other means.[9] Undertaking the ketogenic diet requires a strong commitment from both the patient and his or her parents or caregivers. Because it is a complicated medical treatment that is highly individualized and strictly controlled, it should not be undertaken without the supervision of experienced medical professionals.

References

1. Leppik IE: Intractable epilepsy in adults. In: Theodore WH, ed. *Surgical Treatment of Epilepsy* (*Epilepsy Res* suppl 5), 1992, pp 7-11.

2. Walczak TS: Neocortical temporal lobe epilepsy: characterizing the syndrome. *Epilepsia* 1995;36(7):633-635.

3. Sperling MR, O'Connor MJ, Saykin AJ, et al: Temporal lobectomy for refractory epilepsy. *JAMA* 1996;276(6):470-475.

4. Luders HO: *Epilepsy Surgery*. New York, Raven Press, 1992.

5. Engel J Jr: *Surgical Treatment of the Epilepsies*. 2nd ed. New York, NY, Raven Press, 1993.

6. Wada J, Rasmussen T: Intracarotid injection of sodium amytal for the lateralization of cerebral speech dominance: Experimental and clinical observations. *J Neurosurg* 1960;17:266-282.

7. Rasmussen T: Hemispherectomy for seizures revisited. *Can J Neurol Sci* 1983;10:71-78.

8. Wyllie E: Corpus callosotomy for intractable generalized epilepsy. *J Pediatr* 1988;113:255-261.

9. Swink T, Vining E, Freeman J: The ketogenic diet: 1997. In: *Advances in Pediatrics*. New York, NY, Mosby-Yearbook Inc, 1997 pp 297-329.

Chapter 14

Driving and Regulatory Issues

Physicians often become involved in regulatory issues when caring for patients with epilepsy because these may require medical information for resolution. A common area of physician involvement is certification of driving privileges. In addition, the recently enacted Americans with Disabilities Act has greatly increased the opportunities for patients with epilepsy and other medical problems to challenge restrictions in the workplace, for which they will need medical reports to support their claims.

In the United States, laws and regulations emanate from federal, state, or local government. Those derived from federal government are enacted by Congress and are applicable to all of the states. These usually cover broad, national issues such as civil rights, Social Security, Medicare, and the Americans With Disabilities Act. Areas such as driving restrictions and workmen's compensation are in the states' jurisdiction. Table 1 lists areas of law and regulation by federal and state jurisdictions.

Table 1: Legal and Regulatory Issues Involving Patients With Epilepsy

Federal
- Federal benefits (Social Security, Medicare and Medicaid)
- Military service (VA benefits)
- Americans With Disabilities Act

State
- Driving
- Employment (vocational rehabilitation)
- Family law (adoption, child custody)
- Workmen's compensation
- Criminal justice
- Access to health care

Driver Licensing

Every state regulates driver's license eligibility. These often include specific standards for persons with medical conditions.

In the case of seizure disorders, a physician becomes involved at two points: at the time of onset of seizures and at recertification of a patient with established epilepsy.

Each state has its own regulations regarding relicensing. Table 2 gives a summary of the key points. These regulations are subject to change, however, so a physician must become aware of the specific requirements in his or her state. The area of greatest change in the last few years has been the seizure-free period. In the past, most states required a 1-year period from the time of the last seizure. But because of the increasing recognition that patients with epilepsy do not differ significantly in overall driving safety from the general population, many states are liberalizing the requirements by shortening the time from the last seizure to restitution of driving privileges. Some states have removed the terms seizure or epilepsy from their statutes, and refer instead to episodes of loss of consciousness or control. Thus, conditions other than epilepsy are included in the regulations by implication. Some states also have medical review boards that will grant exceptions to the general rules. Some of these exceptions may include:

- a breakthrough seizure caused by a physician-directed change in medication;
- an isolated seizure where the medical examination indicates that another seizure appears unlikely;
- a seizure related to a temporary illness;
- an established pattern of only nocturnal seizures;
- an established pattern of seizures that do not impair driving ability, ie, simple partial seizures with no loss of consciousness or control.

At the federal level, the United States Department of Transportation has regulations that bar anyone with any history of seizures or epilepsy from being licensed to drive in interstate trucking.

One area of uncertainty is the action to be taken after a single seizure. Most states require a diagnosis of epilepsy before the regulations regarding driving go into effect. However, adults with a single seizure are at higher risk than the rest of the population for having a second seizure, as described in Chapter 4. Should a person have his or her driving restricted after a single seizure? This question does not have a simple answer. One must balance the small probability of a second seizure occurring while driving against the considerable loss of income, freedom, and self-esteem experienced by someone losing his or her driver's license. Unfortunately, the physician is caught in the middle of this difficult decision, and regardless of the action taken, in some cases the outcome will not be favorable.

In most states, the patient has the responsibility to report to the state the development of epilepsy or the occurrence of a seizure. In these states, the physician must counsel patients on their responsibilities, and document on the medical record that this has been done. This preserves the confidentiality of the physician-patient relationship and patients can freely discuss their condition with their physician.

However, six states—California, Delaware, Nevada, New Jersey, Oregon, and Pennsylvania—have mandatory physician-reporting requirements. While the exact terms of these provisions vary, they generally require any physician who diagnoses or treats a patient with epilepsy to report that patient's name, age, and address to a state agency, usually the department of motor vehicles or the department of public safety.

Most physicians feel that mandatory reporting laws may be counterproductive because they erode the confidential nature of the physician-patient relationship. Proper diagnosis and treatment of epilepsy depend greatly on the development of an honest, trusting relationship between a patient and his or her physician. Accurate information concerning seizure activity is critically important. If patients know or fear that their doctors are obligated to report their seizures to the state, those patients may withhold crucial information to avoid state sanctions. That nondisclosure of essential information could be fraught with serious medical consequences to the patient. One study showed that if patients know their physicians would report them, many would not inform their physicians of seizures they had had.[2]

Tort law in many states has recognized that physicians may be held liable for damages arising from the acts of their pa-

Table 2: Laws by State Relating to Driving and Epilepsy*

State	Seizure-Free Period	Physician Reporting
Alabama	6 months, with exceptions	No
Alaska	6 months	No
Arizona	3 months, with exceptions	No
Arkansas	1 year	No
California	**3, 6, or 12 months with exceptions**	**Yes**
Colorado	No set seizure-free period	No
Connecticut	No set seizure-free period	No
Delaware	**No set seizure-free period**	**Yes**
District of Columbia	Annually until seizure-free for five years	No
Florida	Upon doctor's recommendation	No
Georgia	1 year	No
Hawaii	1 year, with exceptions	No
Idaho	6 months with strong recommendation from doctor	No
Illinois	No set seizure-free period	No
Indiana	No set seizure-free period	No
Iowa	6 months; less if seizures nocturnal	No
Kansas	6 months; less if seizures nocturnal	No
Kentucky	90 days	No
**Louisiana	6 months, with doctor's statement	No
Maine	3 months or longer	No
Maryland	3 months, with exceptions	No
Massachusetts	6 months, less with doctor's statement	No
Michigan	6 months, less at discretion of department	No
Minnesota	6 months, with exceptions	No
**Mississippi	1 year	No
Missouri	6 months, with doctor's recommendation	No

* Modified from Epilepsy Foundation Legal Advocacy Department and reflects data as of May 2000. Most states do not require physicians to report epilepsy.

©1996 Epilepsy Foundation. All rights reserved. Reprinted with permission. Latest update available online from EFA: www.EFA.org

State	Seizure-Free Period	Physician Reporting
+Montana	No set seizure-free period; doctor's recommendation	No
+Nebraska	3 months	No
Nevada	**3 months, with exceptions**	**Yes**
+New Hampshire	1 year; less at discretion of department	No
New Jersey	**1 year; less on recommendation of Neurological Disorder Committee**	**Yes**
New Mexico	1 year; less with recommendation of Medical Advisory Board	No
New York	1 year, with exceptions	No
North Carolina	6 to 12 months, with exceptions	No
North Dakota	6 months; restricted licenses available after 3 months	No
Ohio	No set seizure-free period	No
Oklahoma	1 year, with exceptions	No
Oregon	**6 months, with exceptions**	**Yes**
Pennsylvania	**6 months, with exceptions**	**Yes**
Puerto Rico	No set seizure-free period	No
Rhode Island	18 months; less at the discretion of Dept. of Transportation	No
South Carolina	6 months	No
South Dakota	6-12 months; less with doctor's recommendation	No
Tennessee	6 months, with acceptable medical form	No
Texas	6 months with doctor's recommendation	No
Utah	3 months	No
Vermont	No set seizure-free period	No
Virginia	6 months, with exceptions	No
Washington	6 months, with exceptions	No
West Virginia	1 year, with exceptions	No
Wisconsin	3 months, with acceptable medical form	No
Wyoming	3 months	No

** No appeal of license denial
+ No periodic medical updates required

tients. Specifically, if a physician fails to instruct a patient about the risks associated with impairment from illness or medication, and a motor vehicle accident occurs because of the patient's compromised functioning, the physician may be held liable for some or all of the damages.[3] In addition, physicans must clearly document in the medical records that risks were discussed.

The laws regarding driving and other issues of concern to persons with epilepsy are being revised. The Epilepsy Foundation reviews legal issues and laws concerning persons with epilepsy. Its summary of these concerns provides an easy-to-understand overview of current court decisions and legislation.[4]

References

1. Hansotia P, Broste SK: The effect of epilepsy or diabetes mellitus on the risk of automobile accidents. *N Engl J Med* 1991;324:22-26.

2. Salinsky MC, Wegener K, Sinnema F: Epilepsy, driving laws, and patient disclosure to physicians. *Epilepsia* 1992; 33(3):472.

3. Freese v Lemmon, Iowa, 1973.

4. The legal rights of persons with epilepsy. An overview of legal issues and laws affecting persons with epilepsy. 6th ed. Maryland, Epilepsy Foundation of America, 1992.

Chapter 15

Quality of Life Issues

Seizures and the control of seizures engage only a small part of the daily life of a person with epilepsy. Most patients with epilepsy are otherwise normal. In many cases, seizures are infrequent, perhaps occurring only once every few months or even years. Between seizures, these persons have the potential to lead normal lives and be contributing members of society. However, the triple problem of medication side effects, personal fear of losing control, and society's revulsion of seeing a person struggle with a seizure add up to significant social barriers for the person with epilepsy (Table 1).

Employment

Although patients with epilepsy may have average or above-average intelligence, and otherwise be in good health, the unpredictable loss of consciousness can make them unsuitable for some jobs. While there are no hard-and-fast rules, it is generally agreed that persons with epilepsy should avoid workplaces in which a sudden loss of consciousness may expose them or their coworkers to risk or injury.

A person with a history of epilepsy cannot operate interstate trucks, even if seizures are controlled. Also, there are strict regulations applicable to persons with epilepsy who want to operate aircraft. At one time, the United States Air Force required all pilots to undergo EEG examinations and prohibited flight duty even for those who never had clinical seizures but who did have abnormal EEGs. Driving a forklift in a warehouse may also be contraindicated for some persons. How-

---

Table 1
Quality of Life Issues for Persons With Epilepsy

- Employment
- Driving
- Sports
- Cognition
- Personal safety

---

ever, if the seizures are well controlled, or if the epilepsy is in remission (such as after surgery), some of these jobs may be appropriate.

Another issue is working in heights. With proper safety equipment such as harnesses, which ideally should be available for all workers, the risk of injury with seizures is greatly diminished. Thus, working in high places should not be automatically excluded. The same applies to operating heavy equipment; with proper safety devices, this should not be a problem. If a person with epilepsy works on a farm, tractors should be equipped with a "dead-man" brake, a common device developed decades ago for train engineers, which shuts down the equipment when active control is lost.

There are very few office positions that should be denied a person with epilepsy. However, there may be some understandable reluctance to hire someone with epilepsy to work in a position that requires him or her to make a good impression with the public. One of my patients had relatively brief complex partial seizures that might not have been a problem for most persons, but he found them understandably disabling in his occupation as a funeral director. Thus, each person must have his or her specific needs assessed.

Often, employers who are at risk for lawsuits arising from workplace injuries may be overly conservative with restrictions against workers with epilepsy. Many states, however, have specific regulations protecting employers from excessive liability if an injury occurs in the workplace. On the other hand, the physician should be aware that there may be other factors that lead to an employer's discontent, such as poor work habits or poor interpersonal relationships, and epilepsy is used as the excuse. I have many patients who have frequent seizures in the workplace, but are deemed valuable employees because of their excellent work habits. In fact, their supervisors go to great lengths to make it possible for them to continue working.

Persons with epilepsy often need help in securing appropriate employment, and help on how to prepare a job application or how to prepare for an interview. Even when seizures are not severe or are unlikely to have much impact on the work, listing epilepsy on a job application might exclude a person from further consideration. In addition to governmental agencies, the local volunteer affiliates of the Epilepsy Foundation (4351 Garden City Drive, Landover, MD 20785) may have a training and placement program that can assist in finding work.

Fortunately, attitudes of employers have generally become more favorable towards persons with epilepsy over the last 30 years.[1]

Sports

Participation in sports is important for many persons. This is particularly the case for persons in school, where being on a team can be a major learning experience. Unfortunately, many parents and school officials use the excuse of preventing injury to unnecessarily limit epileptic students' participation in sports. This need not be the case (Table 2). A number of successful athletes have epilepsy. One example is Gary Howatt, a professional hockey player who has been an Epilepsy Foundation advocate for persons with epilepsy participating in sports. There is little or no evidence that physical fatigue, such as experienced in strenuous activity, will lead to a seizure. Indeed, one person with epilepsy in my practice runs marathon races and has never had a seizure while running.

Common sense should prevail in choosing sporting activities in which to participate. In general, activities that involve the possibility of significant metabolic imbalances, such as scuba diving or very high-altitude mountain climbing, should be avoided. Also, sports that involve potential for serious injury from the loss of consciousness should be avoided. These include sports in which the body does not have contact with the ground, such as skydiving. Also, sports that carry a high risk for head injury should be avoided. Location and surroundings also play a role. Swimming, if done in a well-lighted pool with lifeguards or others aware of the swimmer's epilepsy, is not contraindicated. On the other hand, swimming in a river or lake should be prohibited. Some years ago, the American Medical Association's Committee on Medical Aspects of Sports published the following statement: "There is ample evidence that patients with epilepsy will not be affected by indulging in any sport, including football, provided the normal safeguards for sports participation are followed, including adequate head protection."[2]

Table 2
Sports and Epilepsy

Permitted Sports (no restrictions)

aerobics	curling	jogging
archery	dancing	lacrosse
badminton	dogsledding	orienteering
ballet	discus throwing	shot-putting
baseball	fencing	soccer
basketball	field hockey	table tennis
bowling	high jumping	volleyball
broad jumping	fishing	weight lifting
cricket	gymnastics	wrestling
croquet	golfing	
cross-country skiing	hiking	

Possible Sports (reasonable precautions)

bicycling	ice skating	skiing
bobsledding	kayaking	(downhill)
canoeing	mountain climbing	sledding
diving	pole-vaulting	snowmobiling
football	roller blading	swimming
horseback riding	rugby	tennis
hockey	sailing	water polo
hunting	skating	

Prohibited Sports

boxing	polo	scuba diving
bungee jumping	rock climbing	skydiving
hang gliding	sailboarding	snorkeling
jousting	surfing	waterskiing

Sexuality and Interpersonal Relations

With the exception of barbiturates or benzodiazepines, antiepileptic drugs (AEDs) usually do not have a major effect on libido. Although AEDs may have a minor effect on some hormones, including estrogen and testosterone, these changes are generally small. With proper counseling, most persons with epilepsy can have normal sexual relations.[3]

The psychological issues of low self-esteem and poorly developed interpersonal skills account for greater limitations. Unfortunately, many children with epilepsy are socially ostracized in school. Parents may be overprotective. Siblings may be unsupportive. The fear of having a seizure during a date is very frightening. Lack of a driving license is a major limitation. Despite these issues, many persons with epilepsy overcome barriers and develop stable personal relationships, marry, and have families. Women with epilepsy and their offspring are at higher risk for complications (Chapter 10) but most are able to have normal families. Breast-feeding is not contraindicated.

Personal Safety

A person with epilepsy lives with the constant fear that seizures may strike at any moment. One survey showed more than 60% of persons with epilepsy feared dying during a seizure. Yet, very few persons die during a seizure. Thus, physicians often do not address this topic, or, if they do, discuss the statistics rather than focusing on the emotional aspects of the question. Persons with epilepsy also fear injury. During complex partial seizures, patients may scald themselves with hot tap water, set clothes on fire from gas stoves, fall in the shower, drown in the bathtub, etc. Severe burns from irons, stoves, and other household items may occur.[4] A physician should be sensitive to these fears, and be willing to counsel the patient in common sense safety issues. Occupational therapists are useful professionals to help in this area.

Persons with epilepsy need to be able to instruct their families, friends, and coworkers in what to do in case of a seizure. Placing objects into the mouth of a person stricken with a seizure is no longer considered an appropriate intervention because teeth may be broken, oral tissues damaged, or the gag reflex triggered. This last consequence may lead to vomiting and the possibility of aspiration pneumonia. Also, it may obstruct the airway, decreasing the effectiveness of the marked respiratory effort that often follows a seizure (Table 3).

Cognition

All major AEDs have some effect on cognition. These effects are usually mild, and usually do not worsen with chronic treatment.[5] Some persons, especially those with inquisitive, active minds, will describe difficulties with memory, lethargy, decreased rapidity of calculations, and other effects. Although many of these effects cannot be measured readily, patients'

Table 3
First Aid for Seizures

Generalized tonic-clonic seizures

The patient may have a warning, cry out, stiffen, fall, and then rhythmically jerk arms and legs. These movements are very strong and cannot be stopped.

At the onset or during the seizure:

- Help the patient into a prone position
- Remove eyeglasses
- Clear area of harmful objects
- Loosen tight clothing around neck
- Do not restrain the patient
- Do not force any object into the patient's mouth

After the seizure:

- Turn the patient to one side to permit mouth to drain
- Continue to observe the patient until fully awake

If the patient is known to have epilepsy, it is not necessary to call for medical help unless:

- An injury has occurred
- Seizures do not stop in 2 to 3 minutes
- A second seizure occurs
- The person requests an ambulance

Complex partial seizures

The patient may stare without focusing, not speak, perform aimless movements, smack lips or appear to chew, fidget with clothes. Sometimes this behavior resembles that of a drunk or drugged person.

During the seizure:

- Do not try to stop or restrain patient
- Guide the patient gently away from harmful objects

After the seizure:

- Stay with the patient until fully alert
- Reassure others that this behavior was medically caused

reports of them must be appreciated. Sometimes these effects can be more troubling than the seizures, especially if the seizures are simple partial events. Therefore, a physician must evaluate the severity of each seizure type, and weigh it against the cost of side effects. Simple partial seizures can rarely be completely controlled with medication, but they do not interfere with consciousness or function and thus do not need to be eliminated.

Epilepsy can affect anyone at any time. In my practice I treat a number of professionals who developed epilepsy after making a considerable investment in careers and life-styles. The disorder forces them to deal with profound changes in their lives. Below are brief case descriptions of patients who have developed epilepsy and are attempting resolution of complex issues.

Case 1. A second-year medical student had a single generalized tonic-clonic seizure after sleep deprivation. His wife witnessed the seizure. The EEG was normal, and treatment was not started. A year later, a second generalized tonic-clonic seizure occurred and clinicians uncovered an additional history of a family member with epilepsy. The medical student had been interested in a surgical subspecialty, and, after treatment was begun, his career was put back on track as the seizures were controlled. Some mild cognitive effects were noted initially; these cleared with change in medication and time. After successful completion of medical school, the patient entered residency training. However, because of interrupted sleep patterns and stressful work load, seizures began to occur a few times a year despite increasing doses of medication. Driving privileges and operating room activities were suspended. Fortunately, the patient's talents and personal qualities were such that he successfully completed a modified training program. Then, a practice routine was established in which call schedules and duties were adjusted to accommodate the possibility of seizures, which have subsequently come under much better control.

Case 2. A young woman had some brief events in college, which, in retrospect, were probably simple partial seizures. A tonic-clonic seizure occurred after she married a medical student. Evaluation was negative, and no further seizures occurred until her first pregnancy. All of the concerns regarding AEDs and fetal risk were reviewed, and a medication was started. She had no more generalized tonic-clonic seizures but she did have brief complex partial seizures a few times a year. These were not consequential and she was able to raise her family and participate in many community activities. During a subsequent pregnancy, AEDs were discontinued, and shortly thereafter a marked increase in seizures occurred. They were better controlled with the reinstitution of medicines. But after her delivery, seizures continued to worsen and she became profoundly depressed. A complete evaluation was performed, and seizures were found to be multifocal in origin, probably related to early childhood encephalopathy and not approachable by surgery. Because of concerns regarding her ability to care for her children (probably overstated) and her inability to drive, a nanny was hired to help care for the children and to serve as a chauffeur. The patient has developed an understandably high degree of frustration, and is in a counseling program and an epilepsy support program. Although she has approximately four complex partial seizures per month, and so is otherwise normal the other 25 days of the month, her life-style, self-image, and actions with her family have changed profoundly.

Case 3. A midcareer physician in a nonsurgical, clinical academic setting had a single seizure. After considerable research on the topic, it was decided to begin monotherapy with a standard AED. No seizures occurred until the patient attended a convention and realized he forgot the medication. He experienced a seizure that was observed by a few of his friends and colleagues. Medication was immediately restarted. He has been seizure-free for some years, but continues to take the medication. Rationally, this person knows that he is unlikely to have another seizure. But the fear of possibly having another seizure has created a constant level of anxiety, which is revealed only to the most trusted confidants.

Case 4. A suburban teenager developed mild viral encephalitis. Before this, he had been active in sports, was a good student, and had a gregarious, pleasant personality. A few months later, intractable seizures began. Despite trying a number of medications, including some in the testing phase, his seizures were not well controlled. He also experienced a decline in his intellectual functioning. He was able to finish high school and move into a group home for persons with epilepsy who had relatively normal functional capabilities. However, funding cutbacks forced this facility to close. Meanwhile, the patient's father had advanced his career and the family moved to a different city. More than 10 years after the onset of epilepsy, the patient is living in a sheltered group home with individuals of much lower functioning level.

These case histories illustrate that the development of epilepsy can have a profound impact on a person's life. However, with good care, the potential of achieving many goals can be met.

References

1. Hicks RA, Hicks MJ: Attitudes of major employers toward the employment of people with epilepsy: a 30-year study. *Epilepsa* 1991; 32(1):86-88.

2. Corbitt RW: Epileptics and contact sports. *JAMA* 1974; 229:820-821.

3. Frazer C, Gumnit RJ: Sexuality and the person with epilepsy. In: Gumnit RJ, ed. *Living Well With Epilepsy*. New York, Demos Publications, 1990, pp 105-108.

4. Spitz M: Severe burns as a consequence of seizures in patients with epilepsy. *Epilepsia* 1992;33(1):103-107.

5. Dodrill CB, Wilensky AJ: Neuropsychological abilities before and after 5 years of stable antiepileptic drug therapy. *Epilepsia* 1992;33(2): 327-324.

Chapter 16

Comprehensive Treatment of a Person With Epilepsy

Providing the appropriate treatment for the person with epilepsy can be a rewarding challenge for a physician. Moreover, proper treatment of epilepsy can be one of the most cost-effective expenditures of resources because it can enable a person with epilepsy to be a fully productive citizen. Most persons with epilepsy do not have a progressive disorder and so can lead normal, productive lives. However, epilepsy is still a frightening diagnosis for a person to confront because of the disorder's negative image.

The Epilepsy Foundation has commissioned opinion polls over the last decades that have shown some improvement in public attitudes but still many misconceptions about this disorder. But epilepsy does not need to be "horrible," as Aretaeus called it. With current treatments, seizures can be controlled in most patients. Moreover, improved diagnostic techniques can quickly identify those few patients with serious etiologies, and then point to appropriate therapy. Those patients with no significant central nervous system disease can be reassured.

In epilepsy, both medical and psychosocial issues must be treated. A person's seizures may come under complete control, but if issues of driving, employment, self-image, and personal interactions are not addressed, total reintegration is not possible.

Effective treatment involves participation of the person with epilepsy in the treatment team. For the best outcome, a physician should be able to provide a comprehensive treatment program involving many professionals in the team.[1] Surgery for epilepsy is best done in a team setting, because many patients will continue to have psychosocial problems even after temporal lobectomy.[2]

Key Treatment Points

Let us recapitulate the key elements in the medical treatment of epilepsy:

- Correctly differentiate between epileptic seizures and nonepileptic seizures (cardiogenic, psychogenic), or other phenomena resembling seizures (syncope, etc).
- Classify seizure types.
- Classify epilepsy syndrome.
- Choose the most appropriate medication based on the seizure type and the medication's side effects, and start treatment with a single drug.
- Obtain blood before treatment for baseline hematologic and hepatic parameters.
- Check blood levels of the chosen antiepileptic drug two or three times in the first 6 months of treatment to determine that target levels have been attained and are being maintained.
- If seizures are controlled and blood levels are adequate, monitor every 6 months or each year for the duration of treatment.
- If a person's seizures are not controlled with adequate doses and levels of the standard medications, refer the patient to a program that specializes in epilepsy. At this point, the diagnosis of epilepsy must be verified, combination therapy may be used, and evaluation of surgical options considered.

Here is a recapitulation of the key elements in the treatment of the psychosocial issues:

- Review the pertinent issues:
  1. attitude of the patient towards seizures
  2. attitude of spouse, parents, relatives, coworkers, teachers, and other key persons toward epilepsy
  3. need to drive
- Develop an educational plan to address the problem areas.
- Monitor progress in dealing with the social issues.

The medical issues can be dealt with effectively in a standard physician-patient interaction. But the psychosocial issues often require the involvement of other persons. Fortunately, much educational information has been developed by the Epilepsy Foundation, which can be very helpful in providing educational and support materials (Epilepsy Foundation, 4351 Garden City Drive, Landover, Maryland, 20785, 800-EFA-1000). Many local EFA affiliates have offices across the United States and are listed in telephone directories. Their staff can often provide assistance through support groups for dealing with the emotional stresses of epilepsy.

Thus, by comprehensively addressing the issues faced by a person with epilepsy, treatment can, in many cases, lead to a favorable outcome.

References

1. Frazer C, Gumnit RJ: How to be an effective member of your health-care team. In: Gummit RJ, ed. *Living Well With Epilepsy*. New York, Demos Publications, 1990, pp 21-25.
2. Bladin PF: Psychosocial difficulties and outcome after temporal lobectomy. *Epilepsia* 1992;33(5):898-907.

Index

Z

Notes

Notes

Notes